THE

INSULTHIN

DIET

The InsulThin Diet
The Lazy Way to Lose Weight!

Dr. Mike Grego DC

Published by Game Changer Publishing
Paperback ISBN: 978-1-7371654-7-7

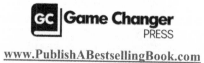

www.PublishABestsellingBook.com

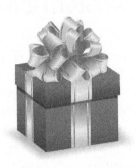

DOWNLOAD YOUR
FREE GIFTS

Just to say thanks for buying and reading my book, I would like to give you a free bonus gift that will add value and that you will appreciate, 100% FREE, no strings attached!

To Download Now, Visit:
http://www.drgregoketodoc.com/book-freegift

DEDICATION

This book is dedicated to our mother and father, Pat and Kathy Grego. They are our number one fans. To our sister, Janine, without her talent and ability to make this book seamless and gel, you would never be able to understand it! And her husband, Terry (the "Rock") Rumker, whose advice is always as solid as a rock! Also my colleague and confidant Dr. Steven Wilder. To Dr. Edmond Zlotea and cousin Mark Tillack for their insights into what's possible and the enlightenment they guided my being.

Dr. Swaroop Nyshadham is a true friend and inspiration. And my grandfather, Patsy Grego, who started us on our journey towards holistic health.

And finally...We dedicate this to the people who desire to live long, healthy and productive lives.

THE INSULTHIN DIET

The Lazy Way to Lose Weight!

Dr. Mike Grego DC

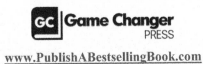

Game Changer
PRESS

www.PublishABestsellingBook.com

ACKNOWLEDGMENTS

The publisher and authors of this book are not responsible in any manner whatsoever for any adverse effects arising directly or indirectly as a result of the information provided in this book.

Grego, DC (20150909)
InsulThin Diet

Important Medical Disclaimer for C G to Nutritional Ketogenic Diet

Dr. Michael P Grego and Kevin Grego CHC Tonda Parham CHC. (hereafter referred to as the "Author") is providing InsulThin Keto (hereafter referred to as the "Book") and its contents on an "as is" basis and make no representations or warranties of any kind with respect to this Book or its contents. The Author disclaims all such representations and warranties, including, for example, warranties of merchantability and fitness for a particular purpose. In addition, the Author does not represent or warrant that the information accessible via this Book is complete or current. The statements made about products and services have not been evaluated by the U.S. Food and Drug Administration. They are not intended to diagnose, treat, cure, or prevent any condition or disease. Please consult with your own physician or healthcare specialist regarding the suggestions and recommendations made in this Book. Except as specifically stated in this Book, neither the author, contributors, nor other representatives will be liable for damages arising out of or in connection with the use of this Book. This is a comprehensive limitation of liability that applies to all damages of any kind, including (without limitation) compensatory damages; direct, indirect, or consequential damages; loss of income, or profit; loss of or damage to property; and claims of third parties. This Book provides content related to topics about nutrition and health.

As such, use of this Book implies your acceptance of the terms described herein. You understand that a private citizen, without any professional training in the medical, health, or nutritional field,

Grego, DC (2015090996). InsulThin Diet: Game Changers Published.

FOREWORD

Hello, my name is Tonda Parham and you are looking at somebody who lost 90lbs in 8 months. When I first started I weighed 250lbs. My size in clothes was 20W. I was a fine big woman, until one day the mirror told the truth to me. I got hurt at my past job and was not able to walk for a period of time. I could not wear a shoe for two years on my left foot due to my injury. That's how I started accumulating all these pounds. So, I got sick and tired of looking at myself in the state that I was in. I asked Dr. Grego could he help me in the state that I was in? He said yes Tonda I sure can. I asked what I needed to do. He said you have to change what you are eating first. I said ok. So I began to eat high fat and low carbs. For the 1st month, I didn't do it right at all. Guess what, I did not lose anything. The second month, I did the eating plan halfway meaning eating right sometimes and other times eating bad. Guess what I lost a little but not much. Then the third month, I did it the way I was supposed to and the weight came off. I know you are wondering what you are saying Tonda? Well, you have to have a well made up mind to change your situation in weight loss or whatever you are doing. You have to get to the point of being uncomfortable with yourself. Guess what? You can! After being in Ketosis, my brain became fat adapted. When your brain becomes fat adapted that is a new lifestyle. I know you are wondering what you are talking about Tonda? All I am saying is whatever you ate before starting this lifestyle change that you thought was good does not taste the same anymore. Your taste buds change! For example: My mother bakes the best red velvet cakes and pecan pies. After being on the InsulThin Diet, one Christmas I cut me a big piece of red velvet cake and thought I could eat it. Guess what? I could not, it was sweet and I had to spit it out, so I gave the rest to my son. So if you want to stop yo-yoing and going up and down in your weight stop die-ing and make a lifestyle change. Today is your day! You can do it! I did and my life has changed and I am loving it!   - I Tonda Parham totally and completely endorse the InsulThin Keto weight loss LifeStyle Plan!

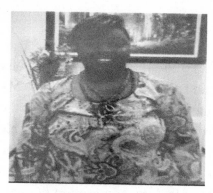

Tonda before and. . .   90lbs after InsulThin Diet Plan . . .

"I wish my life to be, like a leaf, floating on the breath of God"
-Gary Zukav

The information contained in this book can potentially change your health dramatically for the better *if you apply it*. Please understand that repetition is the mother of skill. So, when you want to get good at something, keep doing it over and over and then *you will own it*. This book is set up to be an easy-to-use guide for you to get into and stay at your natural weight for life.

Tonda Parham CHC

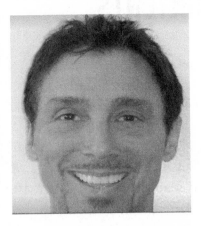

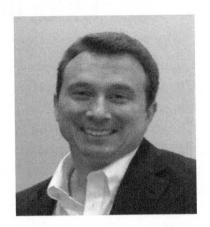

Dr. Michael P Grego   *Kevin Grego CHC*

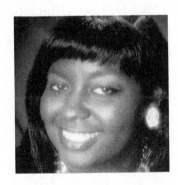

Tonda Parham CHC

"Service to others is ... Enlightened self-service .."
- DD Palmer

TABLE OF CONTENTS

Chapter 1

WHAT IS THE INSULTHIN DIET?

"There is but one thing stronger than all the armies of the world . . .
an idea whose time has come!"
Victor Hugo

Wow! We are so excited to bring you what we believe is the very best version of a healthy lifestyle available today!

Now before we go any further, I (Dr. Grego speaking), have a few disclosures to make:

1. I am a Chiropractic doctor and a Naturopathic doctor and I own a 1 weight loss clinic (The Columbus Weight Loss Clinic).**(Video Tutorial 1)**

2. I treat people that have diseases - not diseases that have people.

3. We use metabolic therapies to help people lose weight and heal people that have diseases.

4. There are Amazon affiliate links contained in this book.

Now that we have that out of the way . . .we know that you have very busy and often times demanding lives, so we purposely designed this book to be relatively short, but hard hitting and packed with simple and useful information (ACTION STEPs), and Video Tutorials (if this is the eBook version) that could and should change your life, for the better, starting today! Also, it is packed with quick and easy delicious InsulThin recipes.

Our mission is to end needless suffering brought on by our Food Industry. And if we are going to do that, then you should understand that:

1. You are caught in calculated web of deception

2. Your weight challenges and chronic diseases will not ultimately get better, until you wake up to some startling facts.

We have a similar mission to Dr. Mark Hyman, who is a functional medicine doctor (Cleveland Clinic). And that is for us to change our food industry, because quite frankly, it causes needless suffering, here and around the world! And so we are joining him . . . because . . .

We believe, like Dr. Hyman, that your food choices, by and large, have been covertly conceived to make you suffer, to make you sick, and to make you . . . obese. All propagandized in the name of a so-called "balanced diet." For example, Tony the tiger, frosted flakes is part of a balanced breakfast. Oh, please give us a break! One of the first deceptions you should be aware of, is the fact that the food industry does not have your best health in mind. Because they hold an allegiance to industrialized agriculture (big agri), which is a 15 billion dollar a year industry. And they use unhealthy and harmful methods of farming. They use unsustainable strategies such as the widespread use of destructive fertilizers, pesticides, herbicides, tilling, deforestation, fungicides and GMOs. Instead of a more natural and healthy way of regenerative agriculture, which utilizes crop rotation, growing cover crops, composting, and integrating animals for more natural and sustainable methods to grow food. Which ultimately would be much better and enriching to the farmer, the land, your health and our well being.

Allow us to explain a little further just how the food industry controls your destiny, when it comes to your weight management and your health.

Directly put,
you are not your ideal weight because of the foods you eat.
And you are eating the foods you're eating because of our food system.

And our food system is governed by rules and regulations given to us by congress. And congress is co-opted by our food industry. How do you ask? By the food industry giving millions of dollars to special interest groups. That wine and dine congressmen and women. To coerce them into voting for "their" particular interests. And that is how "their" laws are made, and that's how unhealthy ultra processed super unhealthy foods end up on your kitchen table.

These foods are then fed to our children and that causes our children to be unruly, more violent, and less intelligent. In addition, they become diabetic and obese. In fact, our kids are so far out of shape that right now 70% of our kids (age17 to 24) are unfit for our military.

This is not just happening at your table, but our entire nation's table and not just our nation's . . . but the entire world's table!

Bad diets kill more than 11 million people a year! And ultra processed food is the biggest driver of chronic illness in the U.S., presently it is responsible for 7 out of 10 chronic diseases. And diabetes and obesity cost our country almost 1 trillion dollars a year. Because ultra processed high carb, low fat foods are the biggest drivers of obesity and diabetes . . .

Now, with over 70% (*71.6 of US obese CDC*) of us in the U.S. being obese.

3

And **86% of Americans** . . .**are OverFat** - meaning they have more fat on their bodies than needed to be healthy.

We know that this is a huge problem and the food system is both the problem and the solution. So we, along with Dr. Hyman and others, are going to do our part, and change the food system . . . *one bite at a time.* . .

We can think of no better time to introduce you and your family . . .to the InsulThin diet.

So, let's get started with a definition of The InsulThin diet.

The InsulThin diet literally means that you are keeping your Insulin
levels very low (15% or less) . . .
when you eat or drink so as a result. . .
you will lose weight quickly and easily by . . .
using your own fat for fuel.

Now we wouldn't be surprised that you are a little. . .

"gun shy" and maybe even a little or totally "Confused" . . .

Because of **All the Different "Fad" "Diets"** . . .

You know the ones that people or the news or doctors or your friends

Talk about or "swear to" such as but not limited too.the following . . .

High fat Low fat No fat . . . .

High protein Low protein All protein . . .

Carnivore Paleo Vegan . . . .

Atkins Modified Atkins and. . .

Clean Keto or Dirty Keto ad nauseum . . .

To clear up all of the above "confusion". . . .

We looked at all of those "confusing diets" we saw a *common thread* in all those diets . . .

And pretty much every other diet on the planet, bar none.

The commonality we found in virtually all diets. . . .

is the fact that they directly or indirectly . . . target . . .

primarily one thing and that one thing .is. . . .

Insulin . . .

Problem is they have NOT quantified a particular number

Or percent of insulin that is appropriate and they have NOT . ..

created an Insulin Cookbook or An Insulin Calculator or. . .

an **Insulin** High End Coaching program . .

Which is easily accessible on your Smart Phone with a Smart Scale that automatically uploads 10 biometrics (once you step on it). . .

to our Insulin Smart Soft-ware located inside Our Virtual Online Clinic.

We came up with all that for you and the thousands of patients and clients we have helped over the last 8 years . . .

And.the InsulThin diet is a Diet that is based on hard, verifiable evidence that when you . . . .

Eat or drink something and keep your . . .

Insulin to a 15% rise (above your base line level) . . .

Or less you will . . .

1 Reach your weight loss goals faster and easier!

2 Potentially keep yourself healthy and dis-ease free for life!

3 Virtually reverse any chronic degenerative dis-ease and fix our broken food industry!

Now you are probably thinking "Wow that sounds great . .

But seriously Just how do you think you can do all that?"

Great question and here is how . .

By using organic, regenerative farming and a . .

"Plant rich" theme not a "plant based" theme.

The InsulThin diet uses plants with every meal . . . .

but they are not the entire meal.

The InsulThin diet uses regeneratively farmed meat and fish.

And the occasional low glycemic fruits, to make the most optimum healthy and sustainable eating plan / diet available today because. . .

It is regenerative for the land, regenerative for your health, regenerative for our country's health and Regenerative for the world at large!

That's how the InsulThin Diet will potentially fix you and . .

Our food system all at the same time.

The InsulThin diet is better and safer than any medication to lose weight and reverse type 2 diabetes. And that is just the opposite when trying to lose weight or reversing type 2 diabetes, by eating high carb low fat, like what is prescribed by our Standard American Diet or S.A.D.

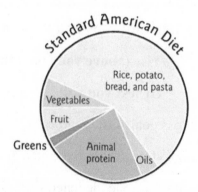

In fact eating ultra processed foods (S.A.D.) causes a constant production of insulin, to be our number one health problem. When it comes to obesity and type 2 diabetes and the resulting horrific decline of your general health and well being.

Fun Fact

We (standard American diet S.A.D.) caused the #1 Vitamin deficiency in America vitamin D deficiency! Because we eat low fat diets, and besides sunshine, fat (cholesterol) is how *we would have made vitamin D!*

In fact, *unused carbs and excessive proteins* cause **insulin** *to be the creator of not one but two of the fastest growing epidemics facing us in the United States today* . . .

Diabetes (type 2) and Obesity (or what we like to call Die-Obesity).

Stated more directly, insulin causes type 2 diabetes and . . .

Insulin causes obesity. [video tutorial 2]

Well, those are mighty big statements.

And by the end of this book, we hope that *you will agree with us?*

To understand our book, the InsulThin diet, you must understand insulin.

So, just what is insulin? What exactly does it do for us?

Insulin is a hormone produced by your pancreas, more specifically, the beta cells in your pancreas. After you eat a meal, the carbs and proteins get broken down into sugar (glucose). Then insulin's job is to ***primarily push that sugar from your blood, into your cells***. So you can have fuel to function. Additionally, if your cells are full of sugar, insulin will ***tell your body to store the excess sugar as fat***.

Thus, insulin quite literally makes . . .fat . . .

What's wrong with that, you say?

Well, nothing on the surface . . .

However, when you constantly consume carbohydrates and proteins. Which turns into sugar. Your body cells eventually get filled up with sugar.

(maximum capacity). So, then your insulin packs the excess sugar into your liver. Then when your liver gets filled up, it makes fat, out of that excess sugar. Through a process called denovo lipogenesis. And gives you a disease called, non-alcoholic fatty liver disease. At which point you develop insulin resistance. That makes your pancreas go into overdrive, by pumping out more insulin (compensatory hyperinsulinemia) to try and keep up with your constant carb / protein consumption. And the more insulin you try to use to push sugar into your already sugar saturated fatty liver, equals more insulin resistance. And more insulin resistance means more fatty liver . . . until your poor pancreas just can't keep up and . . . your insulin becomes refractory (ineffective). And then you just earned a new diagnosis called type 2 diabetes!

We know that paragraph sounds a little technical,

so please re-read it again , for a better understanding.

And, because this is a new concept for you, here is a metaphor to help you understand this new concept, just a bit better. Type 2 diabetes is just like a completely full of clothes (sugar) suitcase (liver) that you just have to put two more shirts in (more sugar), so you jump on top of the suitcase (your insulin) but it won't close (insulin resistance). . . . so you invite friends over (metformin, glimepiride and insulin injections) to help you jump on the overstuffed suitcase (fatty liver). But the extra clothes still wont fit inside the case and they fall out onto the floor (sugar in your urine/blood) welcome to type 2 diabetes!

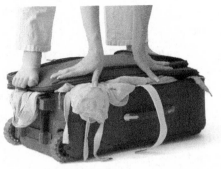

Below is a Flow Chart so you can get a visual on how this works:

THE **FAT** CYCLE

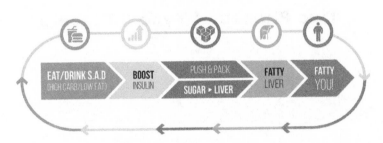

EAT/DRINK S.A.D (HIGH CARB/LOW FAT) → BOOST INSULIN → PUSH & PACK SUGAR ► LIVER → FATTY LIVER → FATTY YOU!

So, understand that when you get up in the morning and eat a "normal" break-fast, a bowl of oatmeal or cereal with a banana and milk. And then wash it down with orange juice or some other fruit juice. That is an enormous amount of carbs, which make sugars (spikes insulin). But that's not all, you snack on some protein bars or chips (sugars), and then you have lunch. Say a hamburger and french fries , with a vanilla shake, that is approximately 98 carbs and 20 grams of protein (more sugars + more insulin)). And then you snack again, candy bar, protein bar or piece of fruit (you guessed it-more sugar). Then you have dinner, maybe a steak and potato, with some pie for dessert (and you guessed it. even more sugar). And don't forget about the midnight snack. . . . a little ice cream or milk and cookies (unbelievable but true-more sugar + crazy amounts of insulin).

Remarkably you are still thinking . . . "This isn't me; I am not developing insulin resistance or a fatty liver or diabetes . . . no way.

Well . . . .

Fun Fact:

A corollary on how to make a fatty liver is like making foie gras. To produce "foie gras" (the French term means "fatty liver"), workers ram pipes down the throats of caged male ducks twice each day, pumping up to 2.2 pounds of grains (starchy carbs/sugars)(S.A.D. standard American diet) making their livers extremely fat. And making yours as well! [video tutorial 3]

Here is a huge study (Whitehall Study) to confirm what we just shared with you There were over 38,000 people studied for over a 10-year period.

Two Phases of Type 2 Diabetes

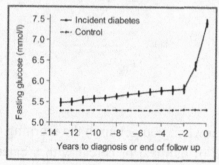

FIGURE 1 Change in fasting plasma glucose during the 13 years prior to onset of Type 2 diabetes. These data from the Whitehall II study demonstrate the elevation of plasma glucose within the normal range

Trajectories of glycaemia, insulin sensitivity, and insulin secretion before diagnosis of type 2 diabetes: an analysis from the Whitehall II study. Lancet 2009; 373: 2215–2221

The top line is the people who developed diabetes, you can see how the top line is slowly (over a 13-year period) going up and up (compensatory insulinemia) over time until their pancreas can't keep up with the required insulin demand. Because their cells have reached **maximum capacity.** Then their insulin can not put any more sugar in their cells and their sugar (glucose) just rockets sky high. Which is when the diagnosis of type 2 diabetes is made. [video tutorial 4]

You might be thinking, "I might be in a little trouble . . .but I don't eat sugar like that. . . . "

Well, negative, if you are not in InsulThin Diet (burning your own fat for energy in the form of ketones) then you are in glycolysis (burning sugar for fuel and making fat + spiking your insulin).

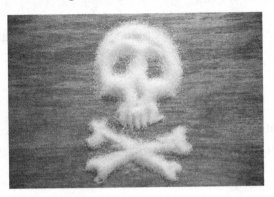

Fun Fact:

Do you know what the number one selling item in practically any grocery store is? The 5 pound bag of white sugar. And it would make sense because the average (American) consumes over 150 lbs. of the white death (sugar) a year! (talk about an insulin spike . . .yikes!)

ACTION STEP

Use Liquid Stevia or Monk fruit instead of sugar. They taste just as sweet and have little to no insulin response or harmful side effects

Allow us to explain a little further, we only have 2 operating systems for using food energy. One is called glycolysis, pronounced "glai·**kaa**·luh·suhs" and the other is ketosis, pronounced kee·**tow**·suhs.

Moreover, you can only be in one of them at a time (Randall Cycle). It's kind of like, when you're either pregnant or not pregnant . . . you can not be partially pregnant right?

So, you see, even if you eat a small amount of carbs, like when you are on a *low calorie/carb diet* . Your insulin will come out, and start making fat. You will be kicked out of ketosis. And as a consequence, you will be back in glycolysis (using sugar for fuel). Moreover, you are well on your way to having a fatty liver, then becoming pre diabetic and finally a type 2 diabetic. As you have seen from the above study.

All because *you are* constantly eating sugars and spiking insulin.

But wait "I really don't eat sugars like that! **I am eating low carb!"**

Negative! . . .

You do eat sugars, "like that", because of a low carb diet (w/o fat) . . .

When you eat carbs you eat sugars. Because you can not use any type of carb (clean carb - complex carb - water based carb etc.) for fuel . . .

Because, all your carbs must be broken down into glucose which is sugar. Then and only then can you use carbs for fuel. [video tutorial 5]

Well, "what if I eat a high protein diet?"

Like in the Paleo, Adkins or the Carnivore diet?

Unfortunately, you can not use protein for fuel either . . . all your proteins must be broken down into amino acids which, in excess, can and do form sugars.

This is done through a process called gluconeogenesis. "Gluco", means sugar and "genesis", means new formation.

Especially if you eat more than adequate amounts of protein.

Right about now you're probably thinking, well then, just what is an adequate amount of protein?

Great question! And the simple answer is,

ACTION STEP

Adequate protein is approximately 20% of your total body weight. So if you weigh 200lbs, you would multiply 200 X .2 which equals 40 grams of protein. And that is your adequate amount of protein per day Capiche? [video tutorial 6]

Fun Fact:

Above adequate amounts of protein, which are sugars. And these sugars have been linked to Alzheimer's disease. Which is now why Alzheimer's disease is now called type 3 diabetes!. Also Diabetes quadruples your risk for Alzheimer's. So, if you don't want to meet a lot of new people (pun intended), you might consider lessening your protein (sugar) intake!

In addition, this brand new study, published March 3 2020, showed when they explored the brain. They found

"Brain networks were destabilized by glucose (sugar) & stabilized by ketones!" . . .

and . . . .

"Dietary interventions resulting in ketone utilization [e.g. ketosis] increased the available energy [and may protect] the aging brain" - Wow!

Side Note

Aluminum deposits were also found in Alzheimer's patients. So throw away your antiperspirants because they contain aluminum. Use natural deodorants like Native deodorant.

"So, insulin has to come out every time you eat a carb or more than adequate amount of protein, making you fat and that will eventually cause you to have a . . . .

fatty liver **(insulin resistance)** = fatty pancreas **(type 2 diabetes)** =

fatty you (obesity) . . .

Are you getting it?

How do you know if you are in danger of developing diabetes and potentially dying in a tortuous fashion, as a result of the deleterious effects of type 2 diabetes?

Make sure you do the following **ACTION STEP**, to find out whether or not you are developing a very dangerous type 2 diabetes...

Because this is the most important check you can do..

To find out if you have too much sugar/insulin in your body!

ACTION STEP:

This is a simple experiment (anecdotal), take your first 2 fingers on your right hand and slide them down your right flank (right side) in the midline of your body (see pic #1 below) until you find your last rib.

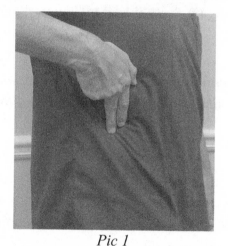

Pic 1

Then gently press in and out a few times. Notice how much tension is there?

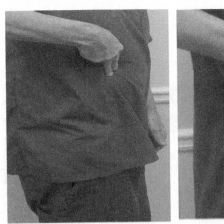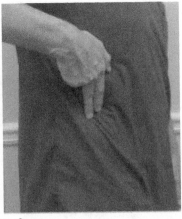

Pic 2

And then slide your 2 fingers forward three inches and gently press in and out and notice if it is harder or softer as the previous spot (pic #2). If it is a little softer than the first spot, then Congratulations (not really) you potentially have an enlarged (fatty) liver.

Because your tissue in those 2 spots should feel the same amount of "soft" tension. So if it's a bit harder at the first spot then your liver is more than likely enlarged. Because your liver should not extend past your last rib! Make sense? [video tutorial 7]

Also . .

Ever wonder what skin tags are a sign of? (pictured below)

While it turns out skin tags are a sign of insulin resistance and fatty liver.

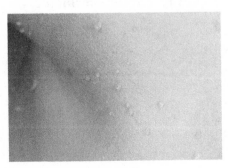

Also, a skin condition called <u>acanthosis nigricans</u>, *which is pictured below, is a good sign that you are insulin resistant and developing a fatty liver.*

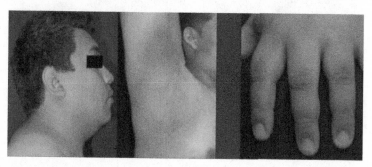

If you wish to know for certain whether or not your liver is enlarged (fatty) you can get some blood work done: it's a liver test called an <u>ALT</u> <u>test</u> *and if it's elevated, you potentially have a fatty liver.*

Now, relative to insulin making you fat, and this is by far our favorite study. Because it's so simple and elegant and yet so very true . . .

In the laboratory when scientists try to grow fat cells in a petri dish . .

they can not grow one single fat cell, until
they introduce insulin into the dish!
"So simply put . . .

you grow fat cells when you spike insulin . . .

so 1 + 1 =

<u>**Insulin makes you fat and you are fat because of insulin!**</u>

How is that for succinctness?

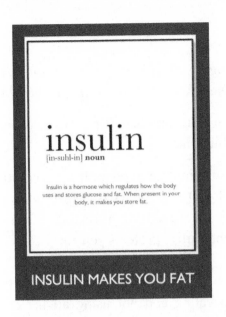

INSULIN MAKES YOU FAT

The title of our book becomes more relevant now yes?

Fun Fact:

Anyone who has been injecting insulin in the same spot for a while, knows that they will develop fat deposits (<u>lipohypertrophy</u>), at the site of the injection.

See below . . .

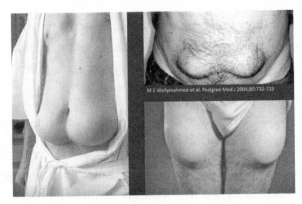

The lumps and bumps pictured above are fat deposits from their insulin injections . . . .

How does that grab you for a "visual" causation?

ACTION STEP

Change from using Insulin and sugar for fuel and use good healthy fats and ketones instead. That's, of course, the InsulThin Diet.

Let's give you one more simple metaphor to help you really understand this very important point.

If you look at insulin like food police, every time you eat ultra processed food (S.A.D.), the police (insulin) comes out. And as long as you stay within the speed limit (eating limit) that is, you use (metabolize) all the carbs / proteins you eat.

You will not get a ticket (fat).

But, if you keep eating and not using all the carbs and excessive proteins (sugars), then you are constantly over the speed limit (repetitive speeding tickets) . . .

The insulin police will then take you to a "jail cell" aka "fat cell" and where you'll be spending large amounts of time, making lots of fat cells (obesity) . . .

for all those speeding tickets (carbs/excessive proteins)… Comprende?

At this point you will have 2 choices:

1. Continue eating the same way, and not using (metabolizing) all your excessive proteins and carbs. Buy a radar detector (food app for counting calories, carbs, proteins and fats).

    This is a very tedious and cumbersome task. More rules to follow.Not to mention extremely inconvenient, especially when your life is already, so packed full of tasks and to do lists! Or…

2. Get a bail bondsman, InsulThin Diet, which uses good healthy fats and your fat for fuel. And then you will be running your car on the autobahn with no speed limit!

- No food Police (Insulin response)

- No "unused" carbs or excessive proteins

- No counting calories

- No making you fat - because the extra fat calories from ketones never change back to fat, even if you don't use them!

Now, which one sounds easier? A whole lot more fun?

We would like to share just a bit more on the "you do not need to count calories" How can this be? We were always taught to watch/count our calories.

Well they, calories can't be counted because your body has no decoding device for calories. *That is to say you have no receptors on any of your cells to measure calories.*

Ergo, you don't need to count them because . . .
you can't count them!

Ponder that for a moment, we will have more on this very important point a little bit later on in the book. . .

For now, let's put your weight into more concrete terms, where the rubber hits the road, so to speak This is where being overweight affects your pocket book Let's look at the effect of weight on salary. Weight affects salary significantly, but the effect is different for men and women. For women, the skinnier you are, the more money you'll make. Women are punished for *any* weight gain (sorry). For American women, a 25-pound weight gain produces an average decrease in salary of $15,572 per year.

Very thin women (BMI < 20) earn approximately $22,000 more than an average weight woman. Very heavy women (over 30 BMI) earn about $19,000 less than the average!

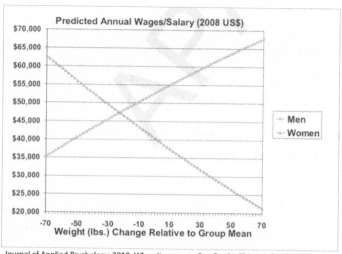

Journal of Applied Psychology, 2010. When It comes to Pay, Do the Thin Win? Judge TA

Ergo, ladies and gentlemen, it pays to be thin!

Besides, being healthier, having higher self-esteem, more confidence, less anxiety, less depression, being thin literally puts money in your bank account!

In other words Being Thin Wins!

Oh, but there is more, much more, are you ready?

Chapter 2

IS THE INSULTHIN DIET JUST FOR DIABETICS?

"Speak your truth and not somebody else's "
Dr. Lustig

Well, is The InsulThin diet just for diabetics? *absolutely not* it is for anyone who wants <u>more energy</u> - <u>less anxiety/depression</u> - <u>better sleep</u> and more <u>sex drive</u>. Sound like anyone you know?

It will supercharge your immune system. Being on the InsulThin diet could potentially reverse virtually all your chronic illnesses such as, but not limited to the following:

<u>Heart disease</u>   Feeling "Crappy"

<u>Cancer</u>   Blood clots

<u>Alzheimer's (type 3 diabetes)</u>   Increased Infections

<u>Strokes</u>   Infertility

<u>High blood pressure</u>   Hair Loss

Erectile dysfunction

Insomnia

Anxiety

Depression

Obesity

Type 2 diabetes

High cholesterol

"Over Fat" (adiposity)

PCOS (poly Cystic ovarian syndrome)

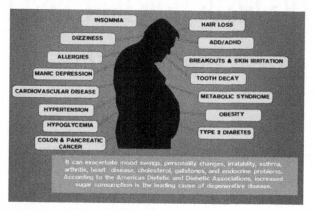

Ok, sounds almost too good to be true, right?

But if we can explain how the InsulThin diet can potentially reverse type 2 diabetes If we look at diabetes as the mascot, for all chronic degenerative dis-eases. Then maybe you will understand at a deeper level what is really going on . .with your waist size and your health.

Then, hopefully, you will understand how the InsulThin diet can help you with practically all the chronic degenerative diseases mentioned above and most of your chronic aches and pains!

First, we have to explain the old paradigm of how diabetes happens, which is unfortunately, incorrect in our view. And let's see if you agree.

The old paradigm of how diabetes happens is based on a lock (insulin receptor on your body's cell) and a key (insulin). And the alleged hypothesis, that this <u>system has gotten "gummed up" for some</u> <u>"unknown" reason.</u>

Consequently, your insulin is just not working. It can't open the lock (receptor), and get sugar into your body cells. Which then causes an "internal starvation" because your cells don't get fed. If you don't treat it, you will die of this "internal" starvation.

Well, there are a couple of massive and glaring inconsistencies with that way of thinking.

Number one, if you look at the picture of the average person with <u>type</u> <u>1 diabetes</u> (pancreas not producing enough insulin) below. You will notice just how thin, frail and emaciated they are . . .

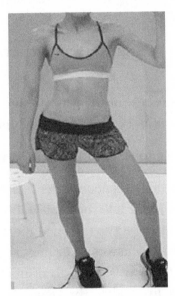

And if you look at the average person living with type 2 diabetes pictured below . . . .

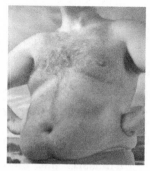

Would you agree with us that this person does not look thin, frail, or emaciated? No "internal" starvation going on there right?

Glaringly obvious agree?

So, that's one huge problem (pun intended) with the present paradigm about type 2 diabetes . . . .

and here is the second enormous (yep, pun again) issue with the old paradigm.

How can your cells have a strong resistance and a strong reaction from the same hormone, insulin? At the exact same time? the answer . .

You can't! Allow us to explain . .

In the present way of thinking about type 2 diabetes they (uniformed MD's-DO's-DC's etc.) will tell you that you have built up so much *resistance to insulin* that you can't get any more sugar into your cells without help of drugs like metformin or prescribed insulin. But, at the same time you have this "resistance" to insulin. Your liver cells, for example, are reacting to insulin. By *taking in sugar (because your insulin is working)* and converting sugar to fat (denovo lipogenesis). And, as a result of that fact, your liver is becoming a fatty liver. In fact, most type 2 diabetics have a fatty liver!

Again, we ask How can your *insulin be resistant and reactive* to the exact same liver cells and at the same time? the answer . . .

They can't ! = standard way of looking at type 2 diabetes = wrong paradigm!

So, you should now be asking, **Well, then, what is the right paradigm?**

Oh, by the way, before we share with you the right paradigm this is the cover of the American Diabetes Association' food choices . .

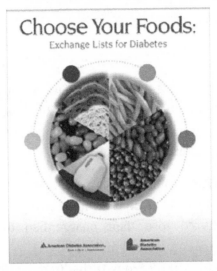

Do you see anything that might be too full of sugar?

And "yes" those are jelly beans in the pic!

Ok, thanks for asking, the right way of looking at type 2 diabetes, is that your . . .

Body cells are supersaturated with glucose intracellularly . . .

In plain English, **your body cells are so drenched and soaked with sugar** that they reached their *"maximum capacity"* . . .

They have reached their limit . . . .

and as a result. . .

You just can not fit any more sugar into your body cells!

That's right, your body cells are literally supersaturated bags of sugar water!

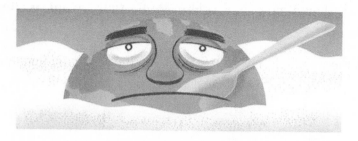

Which are rotting away your body parts because sugar is:

a. Acidic (lowers interstitial pH) - and this literally decays and burns through your body parts. Which in the case of your arteries to **bleed**, and make conditions like blindness (retinopathies) and strokes.

b. Toxic - sugar produces white fat (visceral) which is hugely inflammatory in your body. It lowers your cells voltage which causes cells to lose their charge,then they stick together (erythrocyte aggregation) and can **block** your arteries and give you myocardial infarctions. Which are heart attacks. Or brain infarctions, which are strokes and TIA's. Or rheumatoid arthritis or lupus.

c. Hypoxic - which means it lowers your body's ability to carry oxygen. Then you become hypoxic, which wakes up bugs. By that, we mean the bugs that are always inside you, waiting for an opportunity to have lunch on your body parts. **Bugs** such as bacteria, virus, yeast, fungus and even cancer. These bugs love to breathe carbon dioxide (CO_2) and they suffocate with too much oxygen. So, when you become hypoxic, they wake up and start destroying your body.**[video tutorial 8]**

The name of the disease associated with this sugar "syndrome" is what 's called Lactic Acidosis (static, toxic, hypoxic, acidic blood). And is brought on because of our Food Industry that makes ultra processed food and diet drinks. And if you think about it it is rather S.A.D. (pun intended) dietary plan isn't it?

Fun Fact:

Do you know all the different names for sugar?

75 DIFFERENT NAMES FOR SUGAR

Agave nectar	Dextrin	Maltol
Anhydrous dextrose	Dextrose	Maltose
Barbados sugar	Diastatic malt	Mannose
Barley malt	Diatase	Maple syrup
Barley malt syrup	Ethyl maltol	Molasses
Beet sugar	Evaporated cane juice	Muscovado
Brown sugar	Free-flowing brown sugars	Nectar
Buttered syrup	Fructose	Palm sugar
Cane juice	Fruit juice	Pancake syrup
Cane juice crystals	Fruit juice concentrate	Panela
Cane sugar	Galactose	Panocha
Caramel	Glucose	Powdered sugar
Carob syrup	Glucose syrup solids	Raw sugar
Castor sugar	Golden sugar	Refiner's syrup
Coconut palm sugar	Golden syrup	Rice syrup
Coconut sugar	Grape sugar	Saccharose
Confectioner's sugar	High-fructose corn syrup	Sorghum syrup
Corn sweetener	Honey	Sucrose
Corn syrup	Icing sugar	Sweet sorghum
Corn syrup solids	Isoglucose	Syrup
Crystalline fructose	Invert sugar	Table sugar
D-ribose	Lactose	Treacle
Date sugar	Malt	Turbinado sugar
Dehydrated cane juice	Malt syrup	White granulated sugar
Demerara sugar	Maltodextrin	Yellow sugar

Please take a pic of this and use it next time you go grocery shopping.

So, Sugar causes cavities we all know that. But do you know that the problem doesn't stop there? When sugar dissolves in water, the water becomes acidic (< 7 pH). And that acidity is, what actually rots, more than just your teeth. And for the nurses and doctors out there who are thinking but your arterial blood gas can't go below 7.34 or you'll go into a coma! Incorrect arterial blood gas measures **Extracellular fluid** (called plasma) and we are talking about the **interstitial fluid** (IF) that surrounds all cells, not in the blood plasma. And that number can go as low as 4.5 pH. Now then . . .

Acidic sugar with the accompanying spiked insulin will potentially cause:

1. feet (diabetic neuropathy) - which is the #1 reason for amputations

2. eyes (diabetic retinopathy) - which is the #1 reason for blindness

3. heart attacks - #1 cause of death for people with diabetes type 2.

4. kidney failure - #1 reason people are on dialysis.

5. strokes (cerebrovascular accidents) - 5 times more likely to have a stroke because of high sugar (hyperglycemia)

6. cancer - major correlation and firmly established.

7. Maillard reaction- similar to cooking meat. It corrodes your insides which Speeds up aging and causes all types of chronic disease.

8. White Visceral Fat - this is the fat around your organs, totally nflammatory.

9. Alzheimer's / Dementia - Sugar/Insulin "destabilizes neural networks"

10. Erectile Dysfunction - Makes Mr. Happy sad need we say more?

To name just a few major diseases and that's why we cautiously say

di - a - betes is where you **die - in - pieces!**

More of a tortuous way to graduate (pass on) *Wouldn't you agree?*

Fun Fact:

*The derivative of the name - **Diabetes mellitus** is the exact definition of the disease. It's derived from the Greek word **diabetes** meaning to siphon out / pass through and the Latin word **mellitus** meaning honey or sweet.*

So, the passing thru of sugar, into your blood / urine! Why?

Because, remember, your cells have reached their "maximum capacity" with sugar. And sugar has nowhere to go . . . but pass through your kidneys , your body cells. And that's why your urine and blood have high sugar readings.

So, the actual problem is, in the very definition of the words . . .

Diabetes mellitus . . so obvious to some, and yet still so foreign to others

Extremely unfortunate yes?

One more metaphor - If you had a boat (cell) and it could hold 9 people (sugar) . . . and you attempted to put one more person on the boat.

Well they wouldn't fit (insulin resistance) . .and they (sugar) would fall off into the water (blood/urine). Make sense?

ACTION STEP

Next time you are in your doctor's office, share with them the definition of diabetes mellitus.

So type 2 diabetes is a capacity phenomena a "capacity" issue,

Because your body cells are stuffed full (maximum capacity) of sugar!

The conventional wisdom of the day paradoxically sees that type 2 diabetes as *a chronic progressive incurable disease*. Yet and still, almost every time "they" do bariatric surgery. That is when they do a stomach stapling or a gastric sleeve on a diabetic type 2 obese person, typically within 3 months or less, virtually all their A1c (diabetes test) numbers are back to normal. Yet, "they" (well meaning but uniformed medical/Chiropractic/Osteopathic/ professionals) still preach and teach that "diabetes is a chronic and progressive (incurable) disease" . . .

Isn't that heartbreaking?

We don't know the reason why the wisdom of the day can't get it? but maybe it's big pharma (drug companies) clouding their vision, because of the fact that there is "more money in the treatment" than the cure.

That's the true reality about type 2 diabetes . . . .

and doesn't that make more sense, than a person with an "internal starvation" problem, that weighs 250lbs?

As long as you can understand and use this truth for your health and longevity, we have done our jobs.

Oh, and by the way, we did say at the beginning of this chapter that

"Insulin is the cause of diabetes and obesity" . . .

and *doesn't that statement make much more sense now?*

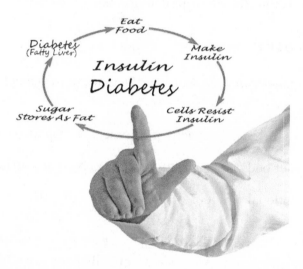

And all this because you have been misled, by the Food Industry, into thinking the standard American diet or S.A.D. , was a balanced and healthy eating plan!

And you have been doing this for how long?

Wow, isn't it really, about time for a change?

Or You can keep doing what you've been doing . . .

and expect a different result but some say ..

That's the definition of insanity!

So, just a bit more suspense, before we share with you the solution.

Diabetes, unlike potentially all other diseases, has the ability to cause devastating destruction to your entire body!

Fun Fact:

For only 2 lbs. of extra visceral (organ) fat, men have doubled their chances of developing type 2 diabetes. And women quadrupled their chances of dying in pieces with type 2 diabetes.

ACTION STEP

Pick up a bottle of Rapid Ketosis because it changes your bad white visceral fat into good brown metabolically active fat.

Also Rapid Ketosis can help reverse "Fatty Liver disease".

Look at the picture below and then answer the simple question:

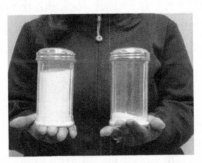

The sugar container on the right is 5% full of sugar. And this represents a person on the InsulThin Diet because they only get 5% of their food energy from sugars they eat. The other container on the left represents a person on the standard American diet, S.A.D., (high carb - low fat) because it's 80% full of sugar. That's how much sugar a person gets if they are on the standard American diet (SAD) *is the person you?*

So, the question is, which person has the best chance of developing insulin resistance and type 2 diabetes? . . .

The "InsulThin" person on the right? Or

The standard American diet (S.A.D.) person on the left?

Pretty obvious, right? the person on the left of course!

Second question, which one has a better chance of being addicted to sugar?

Of course, the person on the left as well.

Yes, we said "addicted" so, just what kind of addiction?

Certainly not like a "junkie" . . . with a drug addiction?

Well, the short answer is a . . . resounding . . . Yes!

Just like a *"junkie"* - with an addiction. Here is why that is so . . .

In animal models researchers placed cocaine on one side of the cage and sugar on the other Eventually all the animals stopped using cocaine and were only consuming the sugar!

Now how is that for an addictive quality?

But they didn't stop there - they then took out the cocaine and replaced it with sugar substitutes (artificial sweeteners) like Splenda, Equal and NutraSweet. And guess what? All the animals stopped eating sugar and only consumed the sugar substitutes!

And then the researchers took it one more step - they removed the sugar and replaced it with high fructose corn syrup. Even though we think fructose is a healthier choice, because it comes from fruit, the animals stopped the sugar substitutes and were all addicted to the high fructose corn syrup!

Point in fact, anything that aberrantly (destructively) changes your body's physiology is a drug.

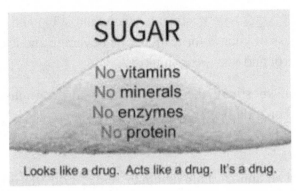

SUGAR

No vitamins
No minerals
No enzymes
No protein

Looks like a drug. Acts like a drug. It's a drug.

Sugar, artificial sweeteners and high fructose corn syrup aberrantly change your physiology and are in fact dangerous drugs!

Quick question, ever feel bad - until you got your favorite diet soda in you?

That's called a withdrawal symptom. And is a sign of drug addiction.

Ever lose self-control? By telling yourself, I'll only have:

a. One diet drink

b. One small bowl of ice cream

c. One candy bar

d. One or two cookies

But, by the end of the day you ate or drank most if not all of them!

Loss of self-control is the major sign of a drug addiction in fact . . .

A 2007 paper used rat research to show that sugar is "addictive" because it induces the release of opioids and dopamines in the brain. *Naltrexone* blocks the pleasurable and sedative effects of opioids and blocks opioid receptors to reduce cravings. Aug 29, 2007

Significance is if we put you on Naltrexone, the odds of you

Going through tremendous pain and withdrawals . . .

just like an opioid addict coming off an Opioid Addiction . .

would be a *"sure thing"* and . . .

AA, alcoholics anonymous, states if you go into a bar and can not drink just half a glass of your favorite alcoholic beverage and leave you have lost self control and you are a "junkie."

And you can substitute the alcohol drink for your favorite go to, comfort food or soda.If you answered Yes! That's me . . .

Congratulations, you are a sugar "junkie"

But, I am not an animal, I am a human being! You all said these sugar experiments were conducted on animals. . . I am human!

Fair enough statement however, the meso-limbic (midbrain) dopamine reward system in the animal study is the identical meso-limbic (midbrain) dopamine reward system in your human brain. [video tutorial 9]

Nice try, but an animal addiction is the same for human addiction.

See the below pic for the addiction pathway in your brain and the animal brain.

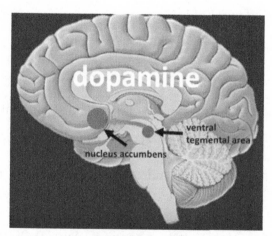

This is your wake up call and hopefully you're getting a little uncomfortable because you realize that this is most likely happening to you . . .

Because ultra processed foods and diet drinks, in all of their forms, cause insulin to come out. And because *insulin* is always around, there are now over 100,000,000 pre and full blown diabetics in the US.

Let's not add you to that huge number.

And if you're already there . . .

Let's do something about it what do you say?

Ready for a better way to live, an easier way to lose weight, a faster way to increase your energy level? And a way to just feel a whole lot better in general?

Ok great! We start by . . .

Asking you a question . . .

If you can't eat carbs or sugars or too much protein because they make insulin come out and insulin makes us fat - then what's left?

Great question drum roll please . . . . .

Getting into the InsulThin diet plan of course with high amounts of healthy good fats and adequate amounts of fatty proteins and moderate amounts of tasty green veggies of course ...

Now, you're probably saying to yourself healthy fats?

I thought all fats are bad for us? . .

They clog our arteries and give us strokes and heart disease!

And besides, how is eating fat going to make us thin!?

Ok, let us answer the first question, fats are bad because they clog our arteries and are going to kill us? Well here is a massive study (pun) (Malmo study) - almost 30,000 men and women showing us just the opposite is true.

The more fat these people ate, the *less chance* they had of dying from heart disease.

Dietary Fat and Heart Disease

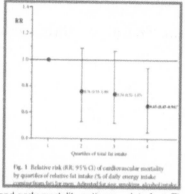

29,098 men and women

Fig. 1 Relative risk (RR, 95% CI) of cardiovascular mortality by quartiles of relative fat intake (% of daily energy intake compaing from fat) for men. Adjusted for age, smoking, alcohol intake.

Dietary fat intake and early mortality patterns – data from The Malmo Diet and Cancer Study J Intern Med August 2005; 258(2): 153-65 Leosdottir M

And then there are these studies from back in the 60's to the 80's.

Study	Journal/ Author	Conclusions
A Longitudinal Study of Coronary Heart Disease	Circulation.1963; 28: 20-31 Oglesby P	1,989 patients followed over 4 years. No relationship of dietary fat to CAD
Diet and Heart: A Post Script	BMJ 1977; 2(6098): 1307-14 Morris JN	No relationship of CAD to dietary fat
Dietary intake and the risk of coronary heart disease in Japanese men living in Hawaii	Am. J. Clin. Nutr. 31: 1270-1279, 1978. Yano K	7,705 men over 6 years. No relationship of CAD to dietary fat
Relationship of dietary intake to subsequent coronary heart disease incidence: The Puerto Rico Heart Health Program	Am. J. Clin. Nutr. 33: 18 18-1827, 1980 Garcia-Palmieri MR	10,000 patients over 6 years. No relationship of CAD to dietary fat. Protective effect of legumes
Diet, Serum Cholesterol, and Death from Coronary Disease: The Western Electric Study	NEJM 1981: 304; 65-70 Shekelle RB	1900 patients over 20 years. No relationship of CAD and saturated fats

showing *no correlation* between high fat diets and heart disease.

And they followed several thousand people for 20 years!

If that's not enough to convince you, then check this 40 year comprehensive study put together by the National Cholesterol Education Program . . .

"recent prospective studies (or meta-analysis of studies) have failed to detect a causative link between (percentage of dietary fat and obesity)" Translation - despite 40 years of trying to link dietary fat and obesity there is still no evidence

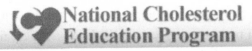

They can not find *any study* that shows that eating fat causes you to become fat and obese. . . .

And the graph pictured below from the NIH (national institutes for health)

Prove just that When we cut the fat out of our diets obesity conversely went up way up!

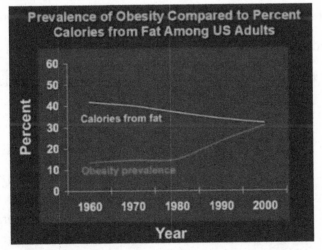

Finally, this just released study on February 25th 2020 . .

<u>LEADING SCIENTIST AGREE:</u>
<u>CURRENT LIMITS ON SATURATED FATS</u>

<u>NO LONGER JUSTIFIED!</u>

And if you just use common sense 30 - 40 years ago we told people fat was bad *stop eating butter and lard and start using margarine and vegetable oil.* And look at what happened to heart disease and cancer rates .

They skyrocketed up to the number one and number two killers in the US today!

Ok, we hope you're getting the point about good healthy fats? And we think the main reasons why you don't like or are afraid of fats, persist because of the profit driven propaganda of one diabolical company. By the name Monsanto.

You see, Monsanto grew enormous amounts of corn in the early 80's.

And wanted to crush its competition, so they ran a massively effective

smear campaign against saturated fats. Because corn oil is a

polyunsaturated fat, so consequently saturated fats were viewed as the enemy (at least from a profit point of view). And so, saturated fats were

mislabeled and unjustifiably labeled as dangerous and deadly.

Saturated fats are still misunderstood today so allow us to clear

the air, as it were . . .

With the following reasons why this happened . . .

Monsanto's corn, in the form of high fructose corn syrup, is in everything from your hamburger buns and french fries to your ketchup and fruit / soft drinks. Even gasoline with added ethanol (corn oil) that you pump in your car. And they are rotting both you and your car from the inside out. Oh, by the way, Monsanto also funded the early erroneous studies that mistakenly said that saturated fat was dangerous.

Monsanto also is the #1 manufacturer of GMO foods/Dioxin/Agent Orange. In addition, they are infamous for putting roundup (glycophosphates) in plant genes. They also produce a neurotoxin (brain damage) called NutraSweet. NutraSweet also causes irregular heart beats (arrhythmia) and brain tumors.

It takes a diabolical company to have such disregard for health . . . Yes?

Which then leads us back to the truth about good healthy fats and how important they are in our health. Healthy fats make up our:

a. Brain - which are 60% fat. Your brain is the most important and fattiest organ in your body.

b. Nervous system - the myelin sheath is covering all your nerves. And is 70 -80% fat

c. Sex hormones - that's right, that hormone that makes you frisky (testosterone), is made out of sterols cholesterol fats.

d. Vitamin D - yes, the number 1 vitamin deficiency in the US. Is made out of cholesterol.

e. 50 Trillion Cells - Yep, all 50 trillion of your cells have a double phospho -lipid (fat) membrane.

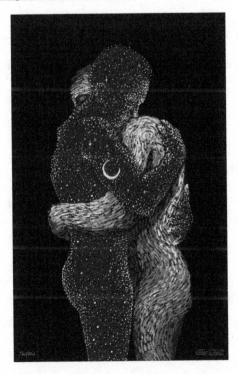

Starting to see why you would need good healthy fats in your life?

The InsulThin diet is mostly good healthy fats with a *lose ratio* of -

80% (+/- 10%) of your daily food energy coming from good fats,

15% (+/- 10%) from clean proteins and

5% (+ 10%) comes from green veggie carbohydrates. [video tutorial 10]

The loose ratio is just that, because when you are fully into the InsulThin diet plan, you are what's called fat adapted (more on fat adaption later) and do ***not need*** to count macros or calories. As a general rule, a good loose macro ratio of 100 grams or more of good healthy fats / 25 grams or less grams of protein / 10 grams or less of carbs is an easy way to think about the InsulThin diet.

Basically, the 10% or so variability is coming from your individual activity levels. The more active you are, the more carbs and proteins you can consume. Without throwing you out of the 15% insulin spike rule.

This Next Point Changes Everything . . . .

More important than any of these numbers
is the 15% Insulin Spike Rule.

Calories don't count (literally) - Counting Carbs is unnecessary

Looking at Macro's is ok BUT . .
the Only Number that really matters is

The **15% or less Spike in Your Insulin levels** . .

When you eat or drink something!

This 15% Insulin Spike Rule is based off the **Food Insulin Index (FII)**

Which were calculated using thirty-eight foods separated into six food categories (fruit, bakery products, snacks, carbohydrate-rich foods, protein-rich foods, and breakfast cereals) were fed to groups of 11-13 healthy subjects. Finger-prick blood samples were obtained every 15 min over 120 min. An insulin score was calculated from the area under the insulin response curve for each food with use of white bread as the reference food (score = 100%).

SAD FACT:

Dr Joseph Kraft was a MD that did over 45,000 blood sugar tests,but he did them with insulin tests as well. And basically, what he found was the normal glucose tolerance tests (GTT) and normal fasting glucose tests . . .and even normal A1c tests are . . .   WORTHLESS!

That's right they are all worthless because if your doctor does not test your insulin levels after you eat - You will never know whether your blood sugar is normal or if you are pre-diabetic or even diabetic. Because your pancreas is pumping out more insulin (compensatory hyperinsulinemia) and keeping your sugar in a normal range . . .Even though it is NOT NORMAL! Which causes your body to degenerate with conditions like: peripheral neuropathy - retinopathy (blindness) - strokes - heart disease and even cancer!

And it is backed by a study that included *every person in the entire USA.*

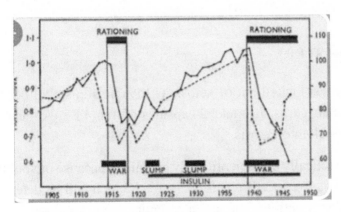

T. L. CLEAVE, M.R.C.P. (Lond.) *Member of the Institute of Linguists Surgeon-Captain Royal Navy (Retd.) Formerly Director of Medical Research,Institute of Naval Medicine*

If you look at the graph above - the lines on the left going up, represent sugar/insulin and all the deaths that occured with diabetes (and its

41

associated conditions - Dementia/Strokes/Heart Dx/Cancer). Then when world war 1 came so did food rationing. Sugar went down - Insulin went down - All the diabetic and related deaths went down! Then the war ended - sugar went up - insulin went up - deaths went up!

To make sure it was not a fluke or coincidence - world war 2 came - rations came back - sugar went down - insulin went down - and you guessed it - deaths went down! So this lifestyle is not just for your weight control Its also for your longer happier life control!

Another Sad Fact:

The reason why you don't hear about insulin so much is because of the fact that a doctor by the name of Ansel Keys was appointed counsel to find out why so many people were dying of heart related diseases. And he skewed the studies to show that it was fat causing all the blockages and artery dysregulation. And ultimately heart disease.

Even though the true evidence . . . disproves that theory.

The politicians and media took the false evidence and ran with it . . .and that's why we still hear that outdated rhetoric about fat being bad for us.

The 15% Insulin Spike Rule is literally a *Life Changer!*

ACTION STEP

If you do get kicked out of ketosis (<15% insulin spike) because you ate too many carbs. Just take 2 capsules of Rapid Ketosis and you will be right back into ketosis.

This is practically and scientifically explained because of your base line homeostatic (balanced) levels of insulin. Which will be determined by the amount of activity you do on a regular basis. Make sense?

Yes but how is eating fat going to make us thin?

When you're in The InsulThin Diet, you use your fat for fuel and you don't make fat.

***Because your insulin falls very low and
won't stop you from burning fat.***

As a result of ***lower insulin***, your body turns fat into <u>ketones, which are
like energizer bunnies, for you to use as fuel</u>.

Thus the InsulThin diet's ability to keep insulin at bay, is the *"secret
sauce"* for you to lose weight when you are eating fat.

And that's how you lose fat by eating fat.

The only reason why you need to have a low level of insulin is for fight
or flight type of emergencies. And because some athletic sports require
explosive movements. Because sugar burns faster, <u>not cleaner</u>, not
better, not longer, <u>but faster than fat</u>. So, it's for when you have to do
heroic interventions. For example pulling someone from a burning car.
You will need an insulin response to quickly dump sugar into your cells
for that emergency *Does that make sense?*

So, other than those heroic - emergency type situations, and certain
athletic endeavors (explosive movements), you will be in a keto state,
burning your own fat for fuel, losing weight, feeling great. And eating
off the InsulThin grocery list, which we will go over in Chapter 4.

We know what some of you are starting to think If I am not eating that
many carbs or proteins . . .

Where am I getting my good nutrition from?

My vitamins and minerals?

From <u>fats</u>, not <u>trans fats</u> (<u>vegetable oils</u>), but from <u>good healthy fats</u>

You have to understand how they calculate nutritional data, that's in
our foods. What goes on the food's respective package labels.

First of all, they are <u>calculated using fractions</u>, you have a numerator
on top and a denominator on the bottom. So they calculate the absolute
amount of nutrients in the food (numerator). And then, they divide it
by the amount of fat (denominator), they divide it by fat because it's so
prevalent and so "unwanted". So if you divide a bigger number by a

smaller number you end up with a smaller number. So, what this does, is bias against the fat (bigger number). That's why you can have a piece of carrot, being more nutritious than a piece of cheese. **Which is completely ludicrous.**

The lesson here is Don't be deceived into thinking you're losing out on good nutrition because you are definitely not losing you're gaining.

You're gaining nutrition, because you get essential fats and essential amino acids when you eat good fats.

The meaning of essential here means, we have to have these nutrients or we will die.

We do not make them; we have to get them from what we eat or drink.

Make sense?

Relevance here is, there are no essential proteins or essential carbs. Because ...

1. You can live without carbs or proteins because fats can and do make glucose (from glycerol) and fats can and do make amino acids from a process involving alpha-ketoglutarate and oxaloacetate (citric acid cycle).Which are types of ketones made from fats. But when carbs and proteins run out, you die.

"We can survive without carbs, but we can not survive without fat. Because we can still burn fat when carbs run out but not vice versa!" – *Dr. Fung*

We believe Dr. Fung sums it up quite nicely do you agree?

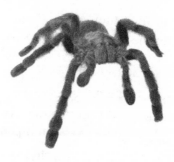

1. Proteins (peptides) are poisonous. That's right, did you ever think about what makes up venom? We mean like the poisons that are in spider bites, bee stings, scorpion stings and snake bites. Well, it turns out that all those poisons are proteins that cant be digested (broken down) into amino acids. The takeaway here is 2 fold:

   a. Make sure you take a digestive enzyme to break down any proteins that you eat.

   b. Think about eating more plant based proteins because plant proteins are in reality not proteins, they're amino acids. Besides, where do you think the animals get their proteins from? Most get them from plants. *See the irony?*

Uh- oh. We can hear the grumbling, in your thoughts out there, especially the men.

"But real men eat meat!" Ok, here is the Man, the Terminator himself, Arnold Schwarzenegger, "milk is for babies " (Austrian accent) and "I'll be back " (Austrian accent) - talking about how he switched from meat to a plant rich diet (sorry the interview can only be heard by people with our eBook version).

So, we are talking about, with you being on the InsulThin Diet,

all your foods and drinks must be
adapted to your response to insulin.

What do we mean?

The good healthy fats, carbs and adequate proteins have to be very specific types that *do not evoke a significant insulin response.* (15% or <)

In other words, they can not cause insulin to come out too much or too fast.

Because, you remember, *insulin makes us what?*

Obese and unhealthy.

But for now, we have to talk about . . . .

Chapter 3

CALORIES VERSUS HORMONES

'You can't exercise your way out of a bad diet.'
Dr. Mark Hyman

Ok, we would like you to read and reread this chapter at least two times, because we all have been brainwashed by the Food Industry, into thinking weight loss and weight gain is simple arithmetic. You know the fabled story, weight loss is, about calories in versus calories out. There are no such things as bad or good calories. Just keep within moderation. So the fable from the food industry goes, all you have to do is eat less and move more.

And a calorie is a calorie. . .right?

All calories are the same right? **NEGATIVE** . . . .

There are *3 colossal and staggering problems* with the food industries "stinking thinking" and they are, the unequivocal and immutable facts that .

Number 1

You . . .

Do Not Have . . .

One Single Calorie Receptor *on any of your 50 Trillion Cells!*

What is the significance of that fact?

It simply means that counting calories does not directly determine how much weight we will lose or gain.

If there are no calorie receptors on your cells there is no communication between your body cells and calories. And if there is no communication between your body cells and calories there is no influence on your ability for you to gain or lose weight because of calories - none - nada - zero!

It's like when Charlie Brown (your cells) is sitting in class, trying to understand his teacher (calories) . . . .

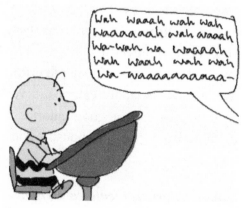

All his and your cells hear are wha - wha – wha nothing! Comprende?

So your body is not counting calories! Why are you?

Number 2

A super huge mistake (pun intended) about calories and weight is the myth that A calorie is a calorie is a calorie But if you eat . .

1000 calories of broccoli and 1000 calories of chocolate cake . . .

1000 calories of broccoli will cause you to lose weight . .

1000 calories of chocolate cake will cause you to gain weight!

Or 1000 calories or brussel sprouts and . .

1000 calories of brownies . . .

One will cause you to gain weight and the other will lose weight . .

Or 1000 calories of asparagus and. .

1000 calories of Oreo cookies . . .

One will cause you to gain weight and the other will lose weight . .

Ad nauseum . . .

Ah But how can this be?

According to the food industry and big agra, who makes our food policies, all calories are supposed to be the same?

That's what you tell you right? **NEGATIVE!**

Because calories are metabolized (broken down) differently depending on your *hormonal response rate*. We will explain more shortly . . but for now these mistruths have been taught to us at a very early age, allowing us to give you one more glaring example of why weight loss is not about calories in versus calories out.

The TV show, The Biggest Loser they all use the eat less (calories in) and move more (calories out) approach to weight loss and even though they lose weight in the short term (6 months or less) they have not and will not, ever have a reunion show. Why?

Because **all the contestants have gained all their weight back!** Why? Because of 2 basic physiological reasons:

1. When you cut calories or use portion control (low calorie/carb diets) you cut your BMR (basal metabolic rate) BMR is the

basic rate at which you burn food energy to survive. And when you lower your BMR, your body goes into a starvation mode. And you will never be successful in your weight loss journey Allow us to explain why let's assume your body has been running on 2000 kcal a day for years. And you want to lose 30 lbs. So, then you are told by "experts" to cut your calories down (e.g. the biggest loser show, uniformed doctors, dieticians, nutritionist, personal trainers, Jenny Craig, Nutrisystem, Weight Watchers, etc.) to 1500 kcal/day, so you can lose weight. Then you will have a net deficit of 500 kcal/day and since there is 3500 kcal in a pound, you will lose a pound a week. And after 30 weeks you will supposedly lose 30lbs Yay Hooray You're done! **Negative.**

You're initially going to lose weight, but then you're going to plateau. And then you're going to gain the weight back you lost and sometimes even more!

Because you have been running on a calorie deficit and your body's not stupid, its not gong to run on a deficit, it can't it will die! *And so will you!*

An example would be you try to take $2000 out of your account when you only have $1500. And if you insist on taking the $2000 out . . .

you are going to jail!

So your body adjusts, it ramps down, your BMR (starvation mode) to match, actually a little lower, than your 1500 kcal/day. Say 1400 kcal/day which means you will gain weight even though you're only eating 1500kcal/day!

And what do you get for all those horrible weeks of suffering and feeling cold, hungry and miserable?

A very upset finger pointing back at you, saying, "it's your fault, because you should have listened to me closer! And you should have had more will power!"

Wow! How crazy and sad is that?

2 All weight loss programs that keep you in glycolysis (sugar burning mode) will cause you to lose valuable muscle mass.

For example when you lose weight through any program like but not

limited to:

A. Jenny Craig B. Nutrisystem C. Weight Watchers D. Atkins

When you lose 10 pounds with those types of programs -

you lose 5lbs of fat and 5lbs of valuable muscle. Which negatively changes your body composition, to a fatter thin person! Or TOFI - thin on the outside and fat on the inside!

Here is a cross section picture of an actual human who is thin on the inside and fat on the outside.

See if you can guess which one is skinny fat (TOFI) A or B?

Here is a hint - the organs are in the center and the white is fat.

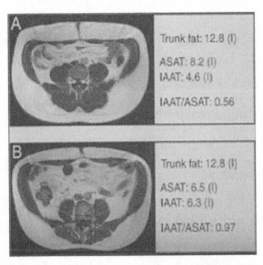

If you guessed B - you are correct! [video tutorial 11]

All the white fat is visceral fat and very unhealthy. A prime example of what happens when you go low carb, low calorie without good fats.

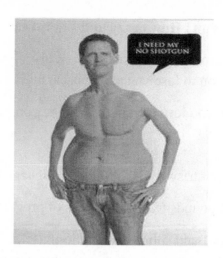

Seems like that's counter intuitive right?

Your weight is coming down, but your body fat % is going up!

Not a smart thing to do is it?

Another take away from the above example, is the incorrect way of thinking that well I am not 200 or 250 or even 300lbs,

so I am not obese right?

Negative it is not just about weight, it's about your body composition. *Body composition is your body fat vs your lean body muscle.* That's the number you want to know and keep track of.

Below is a table of normal body fat %"s.

BODY FAT CHART FOR MEN (%)

AGE																
18-20	2.0	3.9	6.2	8.8	10.5	12.8	14.3	16.0	17.5	18.9	20.2	21.3	22.3	23.1	23.8	24.5
21-25	2.5	4.9	7.3	9.5	11.6	13.6	15.4	17.0	18.6	20.0	21.2	22.3	23.3	24.2	24.9	25.4
26-30	3.5	6.0	8.4	10.8	12.7	14.6	16.4	18.1	19.6	21.0	22.3	23.4	24.4	25.2	25.9	26.5
31-35	4.5	7.1	9.4	11.7	13.7	15.7	17.5	19.2	20.7	22.1	23.4	24.5	25.5	26.3	27.0	27.5
36-40	5.6	8.1	10.5	12.7	14.8	16.8	18.6	20.2	21.8	23.2	24.4					
41-45	6.7	9.2	11.5	13.8	15.8	17.8	19.6	21.3	22.8	24.7	25.5	26.6				
46-50	7.7	10.2	12.6	14.9	16.9	18.9	20.7	22.4	23.9	25.3	26.6	27.7				
51-55	8.8	11.3	13.7	15.9	18.0	20.0	21.8	23.4	25.0	26.4	27.6	28.7				
56 & UP	9.9	12.4	14.7	17.0	19.1	21.0	22.8	24.5	26.0	27.4	28.7	29.8	30.8			
	LEAN			IDEAL				AVERAGE				ABOVE AVERAGE				

BODY FAT CHART FOR WOMEN (%)

AGE																
18-20	11.3	13.5	15.7	17.7	19.7	21.5	23.2	24.8	26.3	27.7	29.0	30.2	31.3	32.1	33.9	34.6
21-25	11.9	14.2	16.3	18.4	20.3	22.1	23.8	25.5	27.0	28.4	29.6	30.9	32.0	33.1	34.5	35.2
26-30	12.5	14.8	16.9	19.0	20.9	22.7	24.5	26.1	27.6	29.0	30.3	31.5	32.5	33.4	34.4	35.2
31-35	13.2	15.4	17.6	19.6	21.5	23.4	25.1	26.7	28.2	28.6	30.9	32.1	33.2	34.1	35.0	36.4
36-40	13.8	16.0	18.2	20.2	22.2	24.0	25.7	27.3	28.8	30.2	31.5	32.7	33.8	34.8	35.6	37.6
41-45	14.4	16.7	18.8	20.8	22.8	24.6	26.3	27.9	29.4	30.8	32.1	33.3	34.4	35.4	37.0	37.7
46-50	15.0	17.3	19.4	21.5	23.4	25.2	26.9	28.6	30.1	31.5	32.8	34.0	35.0	36.0	37.0	38.5
51-55	15.6	17.9	20.0	22.1	24.0	25.9	27.6	29.2	30.7	32.1	33.4	34.6	35.6	36.6	37.7	38.5
56 & UP	16.3	18.5	20.7	22.7	24.6	26.5	28.2	29.8	31.3	32.7	34.0	35.2	36.3	37.2	38.1	38.9
	LEAN			IDEAL				AVERAGE				ABOVE AVERAGE				

1. Body fat charts provided by BodyFatCharts.com
2. Data provided courtesy of AccuFitness, LLC

An example of this (Dr. Grego speaking) is a patient I had several years back. He was only 147lbs but he was the most obese patient I have ever had why? Because his body fat percentage was **57% (+3 really +5 morbid obesity)**. Morbid Obesity means you are going to die prematurely because of the excess fat on your body. And at 57% body fat he was taking more than 20 years off his life literally!

So, knowing your body fat % is super important for your health and weight loss goals.

ACTION STEP:

Go to Amazon and get an inexpensive, but fairly accurate, RENPHO Bluetooth Body Fat Scale body fat analyzer. This will let you know if what you are doing is working (body fat % going down) or not.

Number 3

Gigantic error in our present thinking, about how we gain and lose weight (caloric theory). It has to do with physics and the 1st law of thermodynamics. Which simply states . . . .

The total energy inside a closed system remains constant.

which basically means, if you eat 1000 kcal and burn 1000 kcal, you will not gain weight. This *interpretation* of the law is incorrect.

The law is correct but the ***application is incorrect*** because . .

The 1st law of thermodynamics deals in *physics and not in physiology!*

Allow us to explain. Calories are a measurement of energy when a material is burned. For example, you burn a piece of wood and 1000 kcal of energy comes off it. And then you burn a steak and 1000 kcal of energy comes out of it. Inside your body one of the 2 is going to give you energy. The other is going to give you no energy at all but it will give you a *"splintering"* case of hemorrhoids! Can you guess which is which? Of course you can . . .

Moral of the story is calories do not matter - Instead, what a human body does with calories matters. That, my friends, depends on your physiology **(primarily insulin)**.

Because physiology dictates energy consumption in humans, not physics.

We are human beings not pieces of wood!

We hope that makes sense? [video tutorial 12]

Here is what was supposed to be the biggest study ever, to prove that weight loss was in fact all about calories in, versus calories out . .

The Women's Health Initiative Study, over **50,000 women!**

Women went on low-fat, low calorie diets in their approach to weight loss. Through intensive counseling, women were persuaded to reduce daily caloric intake by 342 calories and increase exercise by 10%. Calorie counters expected a weight loss of 32 pounds over a single year. This trial was expected to validate conventional nutritional advice, "eat less and move more = weight loss".

But when the final results were tallied in 2006, there was only crushing disappointment.

Despite good compliance, over 7 years of calorie counting led to virtually no weight loss . . .

Not even a single pound!

This study was a stunning and staggering disappointment to the caloric theory of obesity.

Reducing calories did not - does not lead to weight loss!

Surprised? well you shouldn't be anybody waking up yet?

So, your permanent weight loss or gain was not - is not -

will not - ever be about . . .

Calories In vs Calories Out!

So please - please - please - ..

Stop Counting Calories!

And start counting ***Hormones*** Yes, that's right **Hormones!**

Weight loss is all about . . .

<u>*Hormones In vs Hormones Out.*</u> .. .

Your body works on hormones. Some examples are:

1. How tall you are primarily growth hormone

2. How much muscle you have primarily testosterone

3. How happy or sad you are primarily endorphins and enkephalins

4. How much sexual desire you have DHEA and testosterone

5. Whether you store fat or burn fat always insulin

6. How well you sleep primarily melatonin

7. How much energy you have primarily adrenaline

8. Whether you fall in or out of love primarily oxytocin

9. How much anxiety/stress you have primarily cortisol

10. How depressed you are primarily estrogen and progesterone imbalance

Because we are talking about weight loss, *number 5* is a super important point and one we are going to expand upon right now.

We would like no, ***insist that you start rethinking*** and fusing with . . .

Hormones In vs Hormones Out

When it comes to you losing weight (permanently) and being happy and healthy. It's all about...

Hormones In vs Hormones Out . . . Ok?

So . . . what weight loss hormones are we talking about then?

Well, there are many hormones related to weight loss . . . but for the purposes of this book. We will limit them to what we consider the top three.

When it comes to dealing with weight loss and overall health. They are leptin, ghrelin and insulin. However, spoiler alert, you will see that insulin is the most infamous hormone, when it comes to your weight loss and overall health.

We are going to start with leptin, which is your "I feel full hormone (satiety)". Leptin is a hormone that does have receptors on your body cells and is directly connected to your weight loss journey. Leptin is released from your fat cells located in your adipose tissues. It sends signals to your brain (hypothalamus) and lets you know you're full. A great thing when you don't want to overeat.

And so it can help you lose weight, right?

Well, what could be wrong with that you say? Two things . . .

1 It takes time for leptin to be released and make its way to your brain. If it takes 15 or 20 minutes for your brain to get and process the signal from leptin. That's a problem because just think about how much food you can consume during the 15 or 20 minutes it takes leptin to reach your brain?

You could have been full and stopped eating 15 to 20 minutes ago but you kept eating Scary, right?

How do you use leptin to help you not overeat?

ACTION STEP:

Eat only half your meal - Stop - go answer some text messagesor emails or look at Facebook - or call your Mom something and then come back, sit down and try to finish your meal. Odds are you won't be able to finish or over eat. So, the delayed leptin release issue solved!

2 The heavier you are, the more leptin you have (because it's made in your fat cells) to tell your brain that you are full and that's good for weight control right?

Negative - the more you eat, the more insulin comes out.

The more insulin comes out, the more suppression of leptin

because insulin dominates leptin. No matter what kind of standard

American meals you eat, you will never feel full, because you . . .

will almost always have room for desert almost always you "just don't feel like the meal is complete without dessert!" - right?

Ever feel that way? Of course you have that's suppression of <u>leptin</u>.

Below is a picture, a schematic, of how insulin blocks leptin . . .

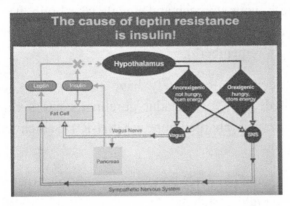

So, when your . . .

"I feel full" (satiety) reflexes do not activate with the standard American diet, of highly refined carbs and low fat. Your <u>stomach stretch reflex</u> for example, does not turn on, when you finish

eating a high carb rice or pasta dish. You could almost always have a piece of pie or some type of dessert after that type of meal. . .and now you know why?

You also have a couple of other satiety safety switches that do not fully engage with simple sugars and refined carb meals.

They are cholecystokinin (carbs/fats), GLP-1 (insulin/sugar) and peptide yy (proteins) and they would love to stop you from overeating but they all only work effectively with high fat - low carb foods. That is why after you eat a meal like ribeye steak and asparagus (w/ lots of butter) and a salad with avocado and whole egg on it . . . you will most likely pass on dessert! Because you **feel full, complete** - your satiety signals are working, properly.

So, insulin is more powerful than leptin, remember what we said in the

beginning of the book *"the most devastating hormone"*

The next hormone, ghrelin, is your "I am hungry hormone."

It is produced in your stomach and signals your brain, it's time for you to eat. And yes, your body cells have receptors to listen to ghrelin (not calories though, remember?).

So, heavier people unfortunately have more overly active ghrelin receptors called GHS-R's (regular ghrelin receptors combined with insulin you get super charged ghrelin GSH-R) Which will cause you to be super hungry . . .

If that's not bad enough, when you go on a traditional diet (Jenny Craig, Nutrisystem, Weight Watchers, etc.), your ghrelin levels increase. That makes you super incredibly hungry, making it even harder for you to lose weight . . .

But wait, there is still more bad news for obese people, your meso-limbic dopamine reward system (feel good and full feeling) takes more stimulation to be appeased.

Take a look at the picture below. . . .

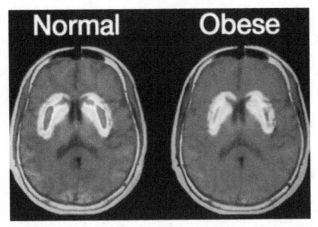

You can see on the right brain scan there are less dopamine reward receptors (darker patches inside yellow). Which means in order for the obese person to get the same good full feeling as a normal person, they would either have to consume more food or sweeter foods and drinks.

Wow, what a perfect storm for disaster, for already obese people!

Talk about having the deck stacked against you right? [video tutorial 13]

ACTION STEP:

Is to eat and drink in a way that does not raise your insulin and/or minimize your insulin response (less than 15%) much more details in Chapter 4 . . .

We save the best (or worst) hormone for last . . . .

the big bad insulin hormone!

You may have noticed the one common disastrous denominator with the above two hormones, ghrelin + leptin insulin that's right!

Wherever insulin is trouble is not far behind - it makes leptin worse and ghrelin worse and you worse . . . .

But there is an exception: if you are a type 1 diabetic = you need insulin (prescribed) because you don't make any insulin or enough insulin on your own. *You can still be helped by being on the InsulThin diet.* And you should be under the care of a well informed health care practitioner in order to find out how you can safely and specifically be helped.

Moreover, if you're sick and tired of being sick and tired, with brain fog, poor memory, anxiety, depression, insomnia, lethargy and you lack libido.

In addition, if you can't look at a pizza without gaining weight

You do not need to use *insulin and sugar* as your primary fuel source

*You need to use **ketones,** from good healthy fats, as your primary fuel source!*

You Need to be on the InsulThin Diet!

Important fact:

Midlife Mortality is where people in the prime of their life (20 - 64 yrs. old) and are dying prematurely. It's rising so quickly and gotten so bad that midlife mortality is driving down our national life expectancy, for both male and females. These people are so unhappy with their lives they are dying early from things like:

1. *Drug overdose (386.5% increase) (primarily opioids)*

2. *Suicides (55.9 increase)*

3. *Alcohol abuse (40.6% increase)*

4. *Obesity (BMI over 30) (114% increase)*

Being on the InsulThin diet protects you from midlife mortality . . So before you think about drinking or drugs (recreational or medicinal) . . . try the InsulThin diet, lose some weight, feel better about yourself and stay here until your time is truly up (God's timing).

By the way we will let you in on a little secret . . .

The InsulThin Diet is not a di – et it's a live - it program based on an **"enjoyable" LifeStyle!**

Because you don't want to die-it you want to live-it! right?

We will let you in on another little secret . . .

95% of all diets fail know why?

Because they are die-its and not "enjoyable" LifeStyles . . .

Your enjoyable LifeStyle is the secret to permanent weight loss.period!

And isn't that the whole point of weight loss?

To lose weight easily and safely and to keep it off for the rest of your life!

Someone just caught what we called the name of this book . .

The InsulThin Diet? What? Why?

Because quite frankly you can not put a lifestyle in a book or a box and sell it. We had to write a book and we have a box (The InsulThin Diet Box) that we sell to people who wish to change their lifestyle. So, don't be confused by the word diet in our book, the InsulThin diet is all about an enjoyable lifestyle.

We understand that in order to make a big change in your lifestyle,

you must find something that you really, really like . . .

if it's going to be a truly sustainable LifeStyle change.

So, it needs to be an enjoyable LifeStyle to you, in order to be permanent.

Make sense?

That is why we have included delicious quick and easy InsulThin recipes in this book.

We have also included a day in the life of an InsulThin person, so you can get a snapshot and the big picture of what a person on the InsulThin diet does on an average day. In hopes that you will find something intriguing and appealing to be incorporated in your new InsulThin LifeStyle.

Now on to what you are going to be using to fuel your body, no not sugar or insulin, but rather . . .

Ketones, which are the fuel from fat, your fat and the good healthy fats you eat. Interestingly enough you do not need insulin to get ketones into your body cells.

And Ketones are more energy dense than carbs or proteins. They are like the energizer bunny They just keep going and going and going.

In addition, unlike carbs and proteins, ketones do not need to be broken down into anything else, to provide energy to your body.

Along those lines, ketones can easily pass your blood - brain barrier (protective shield for your brain) and provide your brain with more energy than insulin and sugar could ever think about providing!

Interestingly Ketones can actually change white inflammatory visceral fat into healthier more metabolically active brown fat.

As a consequence of your brain changing over to primarily burning ketones, don't be surprised if you don't like what you used to like. When your fat adapted, your taste buds change. And you are using ketones, not glucose for fuel So, sugar, pasta, rice, cakes, icing all that *will not* give you that sugar high, that "whoo" -, no siree bobby try not to be depressed over It!

This is truly a life changing consequence of being on the InsulThin Diet. If you don't get that sugar high then why would you sneak around to get your sugar fix or stash your favorite cheat food? Answer . . . you wouldn't . .

Congrats your addiction is broken and you're free from destructive sugar!

ACTION STEP

The Simple Sugar Test

*This is a simple test (anecdotal) - when you are not sure whether or not your fat adapted (keto), just **wet your finger and dip it in white sugar (sucrose) and if you don't taste anything or if it tastes like sheet rock dust** Congrats! You are fat adapted and in InsulThin keto.*

If it still tastes sweet you are not adapted . . . if you are having a harder time getting fat adapted and into keto than getting some Rapid Ketosis Capsules [video tutorial 14]

Because they will help you tremendously . . .

Rapid Ketosis is an exogenous (outside the body) ketone supplement that my brother, Kevin, and I (Dr. Grego speaking) made to help you get into ketosis faster and then get back into ketosis when you get out of ketosis. Rapid Ketosis capsules are available on Amazon.

ACTION STEP:

Go to Amazon and pick up a bottle of Rapid Ketosis because it will not only get you into ketosis faster - it will also get you back in when you get out of ketosis. And as we stated earlier it helps change your white (atopic) disease producing fat into highly energized ready to be used as fuel, brown fat!

This next paragraph is for Clinicians and Doctors Only:

" Ketones are molecules of energy from fatty acid oxidation in the liver and are an extremely efficient metabolic fuel source because they can increase the mitochondrial biogenesis by increasing mitochondrial efficiency at the level of the cell . As you know, the electron transport chain is how the mitochondria makes energy. It is between complex one and complex two and complex three called the semi-ubiquitous site that Ketones have the ability to oxidize Q. Meaning they can enhance the energetic flux of the mitochondria to produce ATP while simultaneously preventing the formation of superoxide anion which is

a highly disruptive reactive oxygen species. Superoxide anion is also a vigorous precursor to other harmful free radicals like hydroxyl groups and peroxy nitrates.

So ketones fundamentally turn down ROS and upregulate ATP production through a more efficient substrate utilization -147 atp for ketones vs 37 atp for glycolysis."

And that's why Dr. Dominic D'Agostino says and we agree . . .

"Ketones should be our fourth macro-nutrient!"- Dr. Dominic D'Agostino **[video tutorial 15]**

Now then, in terms of weight loss and general health you essentially have two choices:

1. Stay in insulin/sugar mode (glycolysis), storing fat and counting calories. Which has been shown time and time again not to work.

2. Going on the InsulThin diet and burning your own fat while simultaneously losing fat and weight quickly and easily.almost effortlessly, by eating foods that hardly ever spike your insulin levels, too high. Because you can eat good healthy fats until you're satisfied and not get fat. Because your satiety mechanisms are working. You will have more energy, better sleep, less anxiety/depression and more sexual desire, all while losing weight.

We would like to share just a bit more on the "eating fat makes me fat" goes well, not when you're on the InsulThin diet. That's because you have what we call "counter regulatory" ketones. This is what happens when you eat high fat and low carb. You make ketones for fuel, like we said earlier and even If you don't use all the ketones, they just become, "wasted energy". In the sense that you did not need them for fuel, so they got eliminated. Some through your breath (acetone) and some through your urine (aceto-acetate). This is an innate protective measure, to prevent you from getting fat when you eat fat. Your surplus of energy was mitigated as "counter regulatory" ketones.(acetone &

acetoacetate) Instead of being stored as fat. Making it almost impossible for you to get fat, because you eat fat.

Do you grasp that? Great!

So, instead of setting yourself up for failure on another fad diet . . .

How about trying a deliciously different
and appealing lifestyle called. . .

The InsulThin diet

Well then, just how do you get into this InsulThin lifestyle?

Great question and that leads us into the next Chapter . . . .

Chapter 4

HOW TO DO THE INSULTHIN LIFESTYLE AND FASTING:ARE THEY SUSTAINABLE?

"Prescription drugs provide a paid vacation,
for personal responsibility!"
Bruce Lipton

We would like to address the sustainability issue first by saying our Creator, God, put you and all human babies into ketosis. And if those human babies are exclusively breastfed . . . they will stay in ketosis. It is our opinion that we should take note of God 's fundamental, nutritional cue and stay in ketosis from cradle to grave.

We are not advocating drinking human breast milk into adulthood. That would surely get you arrested (LOL). Rather, just keep flowing with the original plan and keep eating and drinking high fat low carb (keeping insulin spike 15% of less) for life!

"We can survive without carbs, but we can not survive without fat.

Because, we can still burn fat when carbs run out . . but not vice versa!" - **Dr. Fung** [video tutorial 16]

I know we mentioned the above quote earlier in the book (no we do not have dementia) . . but please reread the above quote by Dr. Fung . . . again. . . because we have all been led astray when it comes to the vital importance of good healthy fats.

The first thing you have to do when getting into the InsulThin lifestyle is to . . .

#1 Stop putting Sugar/Carbs/excessive proteins in your body. . .
So what specifically do you eat?

You eat from the InsulThin Eating Grocery List of foods and drinks that do not cause a sharp rise (15% or less) in your resting insulin levels. So here are the foods and drinks that abide by that rule . . .

InsulThin Diet
Grocery List

% = approximate spike in insulin levels (FII)

15% or more spike in insulin will keep you from reaching your Goals.

*If what you're going to eat or drink will go over **15%** add Fat

(fresh pressed olive oil/ butter and/or take 2 Fiber Caps immediately)

**If you get kicked out of "Keto" then take 2 Rapid Ketosis Caps

1% Pepita seeds
2% Kerry Gold Butter or Clarified Butter (ghee)
3% Black Olives / Green olives
3% Olive Oil - (this is a link to the freshest tastiest highest antioxidant olive oil. Period).

3% Pickles
4% Avocado
4% Coconuts
4% Shredded Coconut
4% Coconut Oil
4% Coconut Butter
4% Coconut Cream
4% Coconut flour
4% Heavy Cream
4% Keto Burger Buns
4% Enlightened Ice Cream (available at Publix)
5% Mozzarella cheese (with 1 fiber capsule)
5% Pepper Jack cheese (with 1 fiber capsule)
5% Goat Cheese (with 1 fiber capsule)
5% Colby cheese (with 1 fiber capsule)
5% Monterey Jack cheese (with 1 fiber capsule)
5% Creps (crepini egg thins available at Publix)
5% Pecans
5% Macadamia nuts
5% whole cage free eggs (1 tbsp. of butter or 2 fiber caps)
5% Eggs (Jay Rob egg protein powder)
5% Egg Yolk powder
6% Bacon (pre-cooked porcine or turkey)
6% New York Strip Steak (1 tbsp. of butter or 2 fiber caps)
6% Delmonico Steak (1 tbsp. of butter or 2 fiber caps)
7% Salmon (wild caught - not pond raised)(1 tbsp. of butter or 2 fiber caps)
7% Sardines (in oil)
8% Sour Cream (regular or Tofutti)
8% Cream Cheese (regular or Tofutti)
9% Rebel Ice Cream
9% Skirt Steak (1 tbsp. of butter or 2 fiber caps)
9% Ham (1 tbsp. of butter or 2 fiber caps)
9% Chicken (free range) (1 tbsp. of butter or 2 fiber caps)
9% Chicken Breast (1 tbsp. of butter or 2 fiber caps)
9% Pepperoni

9% Salami
9% Walnuts
9% Cauliflower Rice (with 1 fiber caps)
9% Cauliflower Mashed Potatoes (with 1 fiber caps)
9% Cauliflower Pizza Crust (with 2 fiber caps)
9% Cauliflower Sandwich crust (with 2 fiber caps)
9% Chia seeds
10% Coleslaw (with 2 fiber caps)
10% Cauliflower Pizza
10% Peanut butter (Santa Cruz crunchy - creamy)
10% Peanuts
10% Cashews (with 2 fiber caps)
10% Buff Bake Bars
10% Tahini Butter (sesame seed)
10% Tofu (with 1 fiber capsule)
10% All Types of Lettuce **(kale, spinach, etc.) (have a salad w/ every meal)**

(must ad 1 tablespoon fresh pressed olive oil or take 2 fiber capsules)

11% **All Organic Regenerative Green Veggies**

(make sure you eat something **green** *at every meal*)

(must ad 1 tablespoon fresh pressed olive oil or butter or take 2 fiber capsules)

11 % Ham (with 1 tbsp. butter)
11% Turkey
12% Pork Ribs
12% Cod Fish
12% Duck
12% Beyond Meat Burgers
12% Sunflower Seeds
12% Sunflower Butter
13% Ribeye (with 1 tbsp. butter or 2 fiber caps)
13% Pork Sausage / Beyond Meat plant-based Sausage
13% Pumpkin
13% Almonds
13% Almond flour
13% Almond Butter

13% Pumpkin Seeds
13% Pistachios
14% Keto Pancake mix
14% Blue Cheese
15% Ground Beef w/fat (grass fed) / Beyond Ground Meat (plant based) (with 1 tbsp. butter or 2 fiber caps)
15% Cheddar Cheese
15% Keto Chips
15% Egg Yolk powder
15% Swiss Cheese
15% Shrimp (with 1 tbsp. of butter or 2 fiber caps)
15% Pizza Sauce (with 1 tbsp. fresh pressed olive oil or 1 fiber cap)
The following fruits are allowed sparingly: (1 or 2 days/week)

Make sure they are Regenerative/Organic + Take 2 fiber capsules when you eat them

Strawberry - Pomegranate - Raspberry

Blackberry - Kiwi - Cherries - Wild Blueberry

InsulThin Diet

Drinks List

0% Alkaline Water Life Ionizer or Evian
0% Rapid Ketosis Capsules - super easy way to get and stay in keto
2% Weight Loss Water - because what you drink matters too.
3% Stevia Lemonade (alkaline water, organic lemon juice, liquid stevia)
3% True Lemonade (watermelon, blackberry, etc.)
3% Coconut milk (unsweetened)
4% Keto Coffee - high fat low carb coffee
4% Ginger Tea (ginger is best for hunger pains)
4% Dandelion Tea (helps flush kidneys)
4% Liver Detox Tea (milk thistle - helps flush liver)
5% Green Teas (sweetened with stevia or monk fruit)
7% Coconut milk/Almond milk (unsweetened)

13% Almond Milk (unsweetened)
15% Solutions4 Meal Replacement Shakes
****Separate the egg whites from the egg yolks (watch this video)

InsulThin

Sweeteners/Seasonings/Bars

Veggie Wash -must use if veggies are not organic!

Life Ionizer machine press 11.0 pH

Stevia liquid	Celtic sea salt	Green onion
Stevia powder	Organic Coffee	Baking powder
Monk fruit liquid	Organic Egg powder	Cinnamon
Monk fruit powder	Sweet Drops vanilla	Garlic powder
Choczero Chocolate	Cacao powder	Key Lime juice
Salsa	Boars head mustard	Cilantro
Jalapenos	Almond extract	Vanilla extract
Italian Herb blend	Garlic powder	Lemon juice
Ground black pepper	Oregano powder	Onion powder
Pork rinds	Dijon mustard	Buff Bake Fuel bar
Sliced Almonds	Taco Spice	Avocado spray
Kraft Zesty Italian dressing	Ranch dressing	Sriracha
Dijon mustard	Garam masala	Kashmiri chilli
Instant Pot	Mayonnaise	Red Wine Vinegar
Feta cheese	sugar-free vanilla pudding	Apple Cider vinegar
Pecan crust	Vanilla extract	Gelatin
Xanthan gum	Cocoa butter	ChocZero Baking chips

parmesan cheese	Choczero bars	ChocZero Peanut Butter Cups
Buff Bake Vanilla bar	Pumpkin puree	Dairy digestant
turmeric	smoked paprika	Garam Masala
yeast-free vegetable broth	coriander	ground fine flax seed
Cocoa butter	tomato puree	ground nutmeg
Coconut Cooking spray	ground ginger	Chile Pepper
Rice Vinegar coconut flakes	ground cloves	shredded unsweetened
Cayenne Powder	sesame oil	sliced almonds
Avocado Oil	Sriracha	Braggs Liquid Aminos
Red Chilli Paste	sweet paprika	coconut aminos
raw walnuts halves	Parmesan cheese	coconut aminos
Real Salt Powder	red wine vinegar	Cumin powder Curry

ACTION STEP: [video tutorial 17]

Click here for a Insulin Index calculator, if you want to know exactly how much of an insulin spike a food or drink has in it. Remember no more than a 15% insulin spike or you will knock yourself out of health and wellness and ketosis. This is yet another reason to get the eBook version, if you don't already have the eBook version.

Now would be a good time to go through your pantry and all your secret hiding places! Throw out or give away anything that is not on the InsulThin Eating & Drinking List. Out of sight is . . . Out of mind!

We would like to share with you all why we choose to use the Life Ionizer Alkalized water machine. Firstly, we hope and pray you are not drinking tap water? If you are . . .STOP immediately!

Tap water is chemical soup, by that, we mean there are so many chemicals added by the aquifer (water purifying plant), such as, but not limited to:

Chlorine - Fluoride - Tri halo methanes - lead - arsenic - PFOA's - Lye

Then there is the runoff from rain water:

herbicides - pesticides - insecticides - fungicides - roundup (glycophosphate)

Then there is the acid rain itself - from chemtrails:

Which contain heavy metals - aluminum - cadmium - mercury - nickel

Oh, and we can't leave out the hospital drugs, when they are outdated,

they go right down the commode, straight to your aquifer, into your tap water. Antidepressants, birth control pills, steroids, opioids there all in your tap water.

If you think your little Brita filter or refrigerator filter will get all those drugs out . . . We have some land next to the Okefenokee swamp, down in Georgia, we would like to sell you . . .

Here is a graph of the United Nations Top 40 Life Expectancy,

to show you just how critical the right water is . . .

List by the United Nations (average for the 2005-2010 period)

Rank ↓	Country/territory ↓	Overall	Male	Female
	World average	67.2	65.0	69.5
1	Japan	82.6	79.0	86.1
2	Hong Kong SAR (PRC)	82.2	79.4	85.1
3	Iceland	81.8	80.2	83.3
4	Switzerland	81.7	79.0	84.2
5	Australia	81.2	78.9	83.6
6	Spain	80.9	77.7	84.2
7	Sweden	80.9	78.7	83.0
8	Israel	80.7	78.6	82.8
9	Macau SAR (PRC)	80.7	78.5	82.8
10	France (metropolitan)	80.7	77.1	84.1
11	Canada	80.7	78.3	82.9
12	Italy (20% above world average)	80.5	77.5	83.5
13	New Zealand	80.2	78.2	82.2
14	Norway	80.2	77.8	82.5
15	Singapore	80.0	78.0	81.9
16	Austria	79.8	76.9	82.6
17	Netherlands	79.8	77.5	81.9
18	Martinique (France)	79.5	76.5	82.3
19	Greece	79.5	77.1	81.9
20	Belgium	79.4	76.5	82.3
21	Malta	79.4	77.2	81.3
22	United Kingdom	79.4	77.2	81.6
23	Germany	79.4	76.5	82.1
24	U.S. Virgin Islands (US)	79.4	76.5	83.3
25	Finland	79.3	76.1	82.4
26	Guadeloupe (France)	79.2	76.0	82.2
27	Channel Islands (Jersey and Guernsey) (UK)	79.0	76.6	81.5
28	Cyprus	79.0	76.6	81.6
29	Ireland	78.9	76.5	81.3
30	Costa Rica	78.8	76.5	81.2
31	Puerto Rico (US)	78.7	74.7	82.7
32	Luxembourg	78.7	76.7	81.6
33	United Arab Emirates	78.7	77.2	81.5
34	South Korea	78.6	75.0	82.2
35	Qatar	78.6	75.5	81.5
36	Denmark	78.3	76.0	80.6
37	Cuba	78.3	76.2	80.4
38	United States	78.2	75.5	80.9
39	Portugal	78.1	75.0	81.2

United Nations World-Wide Life Expectancy Top 40

UN World Population Prospects - The 2006 Revision
2005-2010 Life Expectancy at birth (years)

- over 80
- 77.5-80.0
- 75.0-77.5
- 72.5-75.0
- 70.0-72.5
- 67.5-70.0
- 65.0-67.5
- 60-65
- 55-60
- 50-55
- 45-50
- under 45
- not available

#1 – Japan

#38 – USA
(Just below Cuba)

We are 38 out of 40 just below Cuba. Japan is number 1 and we believe it has a lot to do with the fact that they drink Alkalized water.

So, the Life Ionizer is the alkaline water machine that we use. It gets out 99% of all those drugs mentioned above and then it alkalizes the water. And it restructures the water into a type of electrolyzed water. It's much healthier and cheaper than bottled water. . . and if you go to Life Ionizer water, they will test your water and send you 2 pre-filters. That will take out any heavy metals or organic chemicals you might have . . .

If you are not inclined to use Life Ionizer water, then you can use Evian water.

Evian water is from the French Alps and is naturally alkaline.

Now that you have your list, you can go grocery shopping and invest in you and your health . . . *because you are worth it!*

Don't forget, before you make your grocery list, to check out all the delicious and we mean delicious recipes in chapter 9!

Fun Fact:

Did you know that all bad bacteria, fungus, yeast, mold, viruses and even <u>cancer</u> *can not eat (metabolize) fat . . . but they all love sugar!*

If you don't want a wild animal (disease) showing up at your house . . you might consider not feeding them!

The InsulThin lifestyle does not feed bad bacteria, fungus, yeast, mold, viruses or cancer!

The Most Important Study to Date for Going Keto!

Super Important Fact: If you don't want to catch a cold or anything else!

This meta analysis paper looked at 30 studies over an 18 year period of time. It was published in <u>Virology</u> and showed a staggering 92.8% decrease in infections, by just lowering glucose . . . that's right just by lowering sugar! They said " This result actually supports our hypothesis that infection is tied to glycolysis (sugar burning)".

Which supports our hypothesis:

*<u>**"All germs, yeast, fungus, mold, bad bacteria, viruses and even cancer love sugar and hate low insulin! . . . because they can't eat fat! - Go InsulThin!"**</u>*

Also Dr Mercola's hypothesis in his brand new book: The Truth About COVID-19 - *"All the comorbidities that dramatically increase your chances of dying from the virus . .. are rooted in . . insulin resistance."*

So, if you want to steer clear of any unwanted **viruses (Corona)** the safest and healthiest lifestyle for you and your family . . . this compilation of studies proves ... Sugar is bad for you and Good Clean Healthy Fats are good for you!

Quick question: they used a drug, GD-2, to lower sugar levels, but what do you know that lowers sugar without taking any drugs? . . . . Of course, the InsulThin Diet Plan!

"Make your mind up for what is right and not expedient, and then wash it of all compromise!" - B J Palmer (founder of Chiropractic)

Now that you have stopped insulin from coming out and putting sugar into our cells. We can now focus on the second part of our how to have a healthier, stronger, more vital life . .

#2 Burn off the sugars you already have stored in your . . .

liver, muscles and organs!

And here is how we are going to quickly and efficiently do just that . .

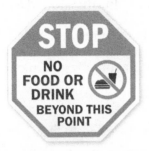

Well, can you guess the above sign is alluding to?

If you guessed, . . . *fasting* . . . you guessed right!

Fasting is the fastest way to get the stored sugar out of your fatty liver (you can't exercise a fatty liver-LOL) and out of your body cells.

And of course fasting is the opposite of eating. So, fasting in the fundamental sense, means there is no food, only water.

And before you say . . ."Ah, I was with you all up until now . .

I can't skip a meal . . .or . . .I will die!"

Hold on a second . .and read the following quotes . .

"The best of all medicines are resting and fasting" - Ben Franklin

"To eat when you are sick, is to feed your illness!" – Hippocrates

"A little starvation can really do more for the average sick man than can the best medicines" -Mark Twain

The above quotes are from some enlightened thinkers , , , Yes? . . and. . .

You know there are billions of people fasting every year, because of spiritual reasons . . .Here are some examples . .

Lent, Ramadan, Yom Kippur and Shivarati to name a few.

Also Jesus also fasted for 40 days and 40 nights.

Then there are health reasons for fasting, some examples are:

Cleansing - Purification - Detoxifying

Your doctor has probably even recommended that you fast before a

colonoscopy, or surgery, or some fasting blood tests, they ordered.

Remember?

Our hunter-gatherer ancestors had to fast. Because if they couldn't kill anything and couldn't gather any food for a while. . . they fasted! Sometimes for prolonged periods of time and they survived, otherwise . . .

we wouldn't be here right now talking about it!

And oh, by the way, you are already fasting . . . every night. When you're sleeping, you're fasting because you have not eaten for 6 to 8 hours! That's why we call it the first meal of the day . . . break - fast . . . surprised?

I just have to chime in here (Dr. Grego speaking) . . .

For those of you out there, that are saying . . . .

I tried keto and it just didn't work for me . . .

I like it but it's too restrictive . . .

I like carbs too much. . . .

It's not something I can do long term . . . . .

While I say, "it's a good thing your body isn't listening to you all . . .

Because you only have 4 to 5 hours of glycogen (sugar) stored in your livers/muscles and if you sleep longer than that . . .

> **You would NOT wake up in the morning!**
>
> **You would die in your sleep . . . .**
>
> **If you didn't go into a slight ketosis . . . . ."**

Fasting is a part of the natural cycle of life. You have to eat, and then you have to fast. Fasting is merely the absence of eating, so you have a period of time when you eat, then you have a period of time where you should fast. You don't eat all the time? Do you?

Oops, we almost forgot, you have been given that misguided advice,

"eat 6 or 7 low fat / high protein , small meals throughout the day.

And snack on low fat - protein bars between your 6 or 7 meals".

And *would you agree with us? That's not really working for you? Is it?*

Our own grandfather (Kevin and Dr. Grego speaking), Patsy Grego, regularly fasted, for health and to renew and regenerate his body. Multiple times he did over 30 days of nothing but water fast. He introduced us to the many benefits of fasting over 40 years ago . . . by sharing stories about how they would fast an earthworms and then. they would regress back to a larva (baby) state (talk about anti-aging) And then they would feed them and they would grow up to an adult earthworm, again . . . and again . .

They repeated the process for over 99 years!

This is a good segue into the next super important point . . .

The 2016 Nobel Prize winner, Yoshinori Ohsumi, won because of his research on fasting. His research on how cells recycle and renew their contents, through a process called autophagy (pronounced aa·**taa**·fuh·jee).

Fasting activates autophagy, which is how your cells destroy viruses and bacteria and get rid of damaged structures, within themselves. It's a process that is crucial for your cells health, renewal, and survival!

Fasting through autophagy, which helps slow down your aging process (increases your longevity) and has a positive impact on your cells ability to regenerate itself. Pretty meaningful . . . right? [video tutorial 18]

In addition, Dr. Ohsumi's research also uncovered how important something called apoptosis is . . pronounced a·puhp·**tow**·suhs. Which is when your cell kills itself. Why, you ask, would your cell want to kill itself?

Three reasons:

1 because *its sick and diseased and does not want to spread the illness*

2 *when its dies, its parts (proteins and amino acids), help rebuild the other cells around it.*

3 *If it's a fat cell, when it dies, it releases all its contents and shrinks.*

  That means you lose weight.

Three super important points . . . especially number 3, when it comes to weight loss . . Wouldn't you agree?

And last, but definitely not least, studies show that you can live longer, increase brain function, boost your immune system, improve your sex life and save money (less groceries - no research link necessary here - LOL) with fasting!

And all the above reasons, ***only happen when you are not eating and in a fasted state***. . . .so, hopefully ,you will stop complaining about fasting and start asking . . . "Well then, just how do I do this fasting?"

Ok, great, thanks for asking . . . there are 5 basic types of fasting:

ACTION STEP:

All fasting methods below are done with alkaline water using the Life Ionizer machine or Evian water.

You must use a pinch of **celtic sea salt (for electrolyte balance) with every glass / bottle of water that you drink. [video tutorial 19]*

Fun Fact:

Dr. Alexis Carrel won the Nobel Prize in medicine by keeping a chicken heart alive without the chicken (in vitro) in a petri dish for 29 years! How do you ask?

By basically flushing **celtic sea salt** and water over the heart cells daily.

The takeaway is , all salt is **not the same**. The right salt can and will help your heart and not hurt it!

ACTION STEP

Throw out your table salt and your sea salt. That's right, your sea salt, if your sea salt is stark white and doesn't have any color to it . . . it's bleached and only contains sodium and chloride which is table salt!

Get a bag of Celtic sea salt.

Here are the 5 types of Fasting:

1 IF or Intermittent Fasting.

This is where you pick a window of time to eat (eating window). Typically it's 4 or 5 hours. So, let's say you chose a 5 hour eating window from 12 to 5 (could also be 1pm to 6pm or 11am to 4pm etc.). So when you wake up - you skip breakfast and your 1st meal is at 12pm and your last meal is at 5 pm. That means you are intermittently fasting

(IF) (no food just alkalized/alkaline water) (Life Ionizer or Evian) and celtic sea salt for 19 hours. And you are eating for 5 hours (12pm to 5pm) . . .do you follow?

[video tutorial 20]

This type of fasting is great for everyone on InsulThin Diet plan

2 Short Term Fasting

This is just as the name implies, a shorter time, fasting for 1 to 4 days.

So you would just drink alkalized/alkaline water (Life Ionizer or Evian) with a pinch of Celtic sea salt. To keep your electrolytes balanced.

On the fourth day you may want to break your fast with a fresh spinach or kale salad, with olive oil/apple cider vinegar dressing. Or eat something fresh and raw with high fat and low carb content. Check out the salad section in chapter 9.

This type of fasting is great for some of you with moderate amounts of sugar stored in your liver and body cells.

ACTION STEP:

Just how much alkalized/alkaline water, Life Ionizer or Evian, *should you be drinking a day?*

The general rule is half your bodyweight in ounces. So if you weigh 200 lbs., you should drink at least 100 oz a day. And just add a pinch of celtic sea salt with each glass of your alkalized water.

3 Long Term Fasting:

*Before starting a long term fast, we recommend getting checked by a well informed Health Care Practitioner.

You might consider reaching out to us by going to our Webinar . . Here.

Just as the name implies, long term is any fast over 4 days. You might be wondering why over 4 days? And, isn't long term fasting harder?

I will need more will power . . .right?

Negative, around 4 days is when your ghrelin turns down and that is your "I am hungry hormone", remember?

And leptin turns up (your "I am full hormone").

Significance is, you are not as hungry with a longer fast..

So, the answer to the question of "will it be harder to do, because its longer?" Negative, it is potentially easier to do a longer fast, because the hunger pains have significantly diminished and your mind becomes more clear. Ketones burn cleaner (< free radicals) less cloudy exhaust = less cloudy mind) and your energy levels are typically up, because your burning your fat and your fat has 225% more energy per kCal than sugar or carbs or protein.

Furthermore . . .you have what's called counter regulatory hormones. They come out when you fast, for long periods of time to "counter" the effects of low insulin. They are hormones like growth hormone, nor-adrenaline, and cortisol. These hormones are neuroprotective (protect your brain) and protein sparing (keep your muscles from atrophying) and upregulate your sympathetic nervous system (which keeps your senses keen and energy high).

Fun Fact:

Ginger tea would be a great help to you, when you are fasting. Because it has catechins (powerful antioxidants) which decrease ghrelin (the "growl" in your stomach). Which will help with cravings and hunger pains. It also has phosphodiesterase inhibitors which will increase adrenaline and give you extra energy!

Other really important reasons to do a longer term fast are, the apoptosis (cell death to feed other cells and lose weight) and autophagy (cleaning inside of your cells) that are more pronounced with a longer fast.

Those beneficial processes typically do not start happening until you get past the fourth day of fasting.

This type of fast is typically what's needed to reverse fatty liver diseases.

How do you know when to break or stop the fast. . .?

While it's really pretty simple . . .

When you get hungry, again . . . how's that for simplicity?

ACTION STEP:

How do you know if you are really hungry and ready to stop your fast? Just drink a glass (20zs) of alkalized/alkaline water (with a pinch of celtic sea salt) and wait 10 minutes. If you are really truly hungry you will still be hungry after drinking the water. Or you just might be dehydrated, because the <u>thirst center is right next to your hunger center in the brain</u> *(hypothalamus). And sometimes those signals get crossed.*

Remember to break this fast, never use heavy food like meats or cheese. Break them with a fresh green smoothie for the 1st day and then the second day, add salads, like kale or spinach, with olive oil and apple cider vinegar dressing. Again, check out chapter 8 for some savory salad recipes.

This type of fasting would be for people with severe amounts of sugar stored in their liver and body cells. People with metabolic diseases, such as type 2 diabetes, high blood pressure, high cholesterol, heart disease and cancer.

Also, (Dr. Grego speaking), we have found that generally people's tumors don't start shrinking until their sugars are less than 70mg/dl. And that almost always requires a longer term fast.

*If you have any severe reaction like but not limited to the following:

migraines - vomiting - nausea - shaking - diarrhea - constipation

You are most likely having a herxheimer reaction (too many toxins coming out of your body too quickly) . . but to err on the side of caution . .

Stop your fast and contact your informed health care professional immediately.

4 OMAD or One Meal a Day

This is typically what a "keto" or InsulThin Keto person would do, just

because It's what just seems to happen . . .naturally. Because with the

Keto people's lifestyle is so much more energy and vitality.

Eating OMAD means your cutting out the prep and eating time for 2

meals. And with no need for naps or breaks, you have just found those

extra hours that you need in a day to get done what you couldn't get done

before. Eating only one meal a day, you will not miss the other meals.

because as long as you have fat on your body you have a

refrigerator full of food, at your constant disposal.

And besides, who couldn't use a few extra hours in a day . . . right?

This type of fast would be for people in the InsulThin lifestyle.

Fun Fact:

Herschel Walker, Heisman trophy winner, only eats one meal a day (OMAD). He is 6' 1" tall and weighs 220lbs. He does a 1000 chin ups and 1000 push ups and 1000 sit ups a day. And has been doing this for years!

5 Dry Fasting

Dry fasting is a more advanced form of fasting. It is as the name dictates,

no water or food. Why would you want to do this?

To give every system in your body a chance to rest and reset.

When you don't drink or eat, your kidneys, liver, intestines can all rest and

reset themselves.. . .

We recommend a 24 hour dry fast. Make sure you are well hydrated

before you start this type of fast.

You would wake up for example at 7am . . no eating or drinking until 7 am

the next day.

If you chose to do more than a 24 hour dry fast,

- We would highly recommend getting with your informed healthcare professional first.

But, if I fast, I am not going to have enough energy! And I am going to lose valuable muscle (sarcopenia) if I fast too long! . . .

Negative . . .remember, you have counter regulatory hormones. They come out when you fast for long periods of time to "counter" the effects of starvation (low insulin). So . . . .

God put these counter regulatory hormones inside you because, remember when we were talking about our hunter gatherer ancestors? We said they might not kill or gather anything to eat . . . and so they fasted, sometimes for very long periods of time. So they couldn't just sit there and use their Uber eats or Waiter Apps (LOL) . . because they were too tired, exhausted or weak to catch animals . . . no, they did not lose a step or lose muscle and they had all the energy and alertness they needed to go get food . . . and . . . So will you!

Fun Fact:

Most of the top critically important pathways that your body communicates within itself, to achieve weight loss and vibrant health (homeostasis) are turned on (upregulated) during fasting. Some of the more important ones worth mentioning are: [video tutorial 21]

BDNF - *Which stands for brain derived neurotrophic factor. What this does for you, is like fertilizer for your brain. It keeps from meeting people, you already know and asking them, "who are you?" (Alzheimer's/dementia) You produce a lot more of this* brain fertilizer *when you are in a fasted state.*

PGC-1 Alpha - *increases your cells* energy (mitochondrial genesis) *Plays a huge role in digesting and eliminating fat (lipolysis) Helps eliminate sugar from your cells.*

Sirtuin Pathway - *dramatically helps control insulin and sugar metabolism Anti-aging. Anti-inflammatory*

AMPk Pathway - *increases your ability to break down fat so it can be made into ketones (hepatic ketogenesis). Anti-inflammatory.*

mTOR Pathway - *is turned on/off during fasting which allows for deeper* cleaning and detoxifying of your bodies cells (autophagy) *which potentially leads to a* longer life *for you!*

Circadian rhythms - these set your times for sleeping and waking. And they get reset for a deeper, more restful regenerative sleep.

Mitochondria dysfunction + Heteroplasmy - mitochondria are the energy exchange part of your cells. When they don't have enough energy you get sick and diseased. Fasting resets and heals your Mitochondria.

Interesting fact, *Angus Barbieri, has the world record for the longest fast.*

He fasted for 382 days! On just tea, coffee, soda water and vitamins, living at home in Tayport, Scotland, and frequently visiting Maryfield

*Hospital for medical evaluations. He lost 276 pounds (125 kg) and set a record for the longest **fast**.*

And you think you go a day without eating . . shame on you!

Now, this is a good time to talk about how to help type 2 diabetes.

If you or someone you know is a type 2 diabetic and on medication(s).

You or they must work with an informed healthcare professional (MD - DC - ND - DO etc.) that understands keto and fasting. Because you will have to scale down your medications properly as well as simultaneously upping your ketones. So you will have a safe transition from glycolysis (sugar burning) into ketosis (fat burning).

If the transition from glycolysis to ketosis is done properly (by an informed health care professional), it should take somewhere between 3 weeks to 3 months, for a typical type 2 diabetic to be reversed. It could be longer, based on the level of sugar saturation (insulin resistance) in your or their liver and body cells.

Contraindications for fasting:

**Fasting is contraindicated for Pregnant women - Children and Malnourished people

***If you have a serious condition such as type 1 or 2 diabetes work with your informed health professional before starting a fast

****If you do not have a gallbladder consult an informed health professional before starting a fast.

Now, we would be remiss if we did not mention weight lifting . .

Why is weight lifting so important and what's in it for you?

Great questions and let us ask you a question?

Is your body fat over 25%?

What's that? . . . You don't have a Dexa machine or calipers or a saltwater tank to measure your body fat. . .

Well that's ok . . . take your shirt off (in private) and look in the mirror. We call it the mirror of truth . . because, it won't lie to you . . unlike your spouse or significant other, who might have to, in order to keep the peace! - LOL!

If you don't like what you see in the mirror of truth . . .

Your body fat % is over 25% . . . and . . . . you need . . .to build muscle.

So, here is the question . . . to build lean body muscle you either need to . .

    A. Walk more and do more cardio? . . . or . .

    B. Do resistance training with weights?

If you said B . . .Then you are correct!

If all you do is walk around or use the <u>treadmill</u>, they will only cause you to lose valuable muscle, it will not increase it!

Weight training is how you change your body composition It increases your lean body muscle, and it decreases body fat. Weight training has 3 major positive effects:

1. <u>Irison</u>- is a powerful fat burning hormone released when weight training.. That burns fat even after you finish lifting. And helps keep insulin at bay by quickly burning excess sugar.

2. <u>Increases your BMR</u> (basal metabolic rate) - this is the rate at which you use energy. With BMR increased you can literally burn fat while you sleep

3. Your <u>Cell Voltage increase</u>s - your muscles are piezoelectric. That basically means your muscles are like quartz crystals. And when you squeeze crystals (muscle contraction) you get voltage (energy). And the more energy you have inside your cells, the more energy your cells have to heal and repair.

What are some of the other benefits of lifting weights?

Well, lifting weights is considered the new fountain of youth . . a 2007 study took a group of seniors, men and women, over the age of 65. And changed nothing but adding in 2 days of moderate weight training. And at the end of just 6 weeks they had . . .

*increased strength by 50%

*increased growth hormone

*increased sex hormones

*increased energy

*increased libido

*decreased stress and anxiety

Does that sound appealing to anyone?

Great, now how do you lift weights correctly?

Well what's that you say, "I don't want to get too bulky or to muscled up and look like those men and women on the bodybuilding stage!"

Ok . . Let's address the last part first . . .

"I don't want to look too "muscled up" . . Ha ha . Sorry we don't mean to laugh but . . .you can not look too muscled up, like those men and women on stage . . . because 99% of them are on performance enhancing drugs (steroids, growth hormone) and lots of them! . . So, you will not use performance enhancing drugs. Therefore, you will not be too "muscled up."

Now then, how do you lift weights correctly?

How to Lift Weight Correctly

1st Warm Up with Correct Breathing [video tutorial 22]

Always breathe in thru your nose and out more slowly, thru your mouth.

2nd Continue Warming Up with Yoga Stretches

If you can't click on the link, then go to YouTube and type in "DDP morning yoga." And click on the video. It's only 5 minutes long.

3rd Warm Up with just the weight of the bar and then use these

Core Weight Training Principles:

A. Warm up sufficiently- the older you are - the longer you need to warm up.

B. Breathe correctly - breathe out on the contraction of the muscle

C. Time under Tension [video tutorial 23] your muscle does not know how much weight you're training with . . . muscle only knows tension and time under that tension. . . like the tension in a bad relationship . . Do you remember?

D. Muscle Confusion [video tutorial 24]

- always change reps, sets, cadence and never lock out (full extension). Because your nervous system will have to adapt and your gains will be fully expressed. Arnold Schwarzenegger has a great quote about not locking out on any exercise. *"We are training muscles . . not joints!"*(Austrian accent) and *"quick . . get to the chopper . . "*(sorry couldn't resist).

Meaning, when weight training, ***do not ever lock out your arms or legs.*** Because then you will keep constant tension on the muscle, and not overload and possibly injure your joints. Make sense?

You will need to do weight training 3 times a week to change your body composition. So that your body fat % will eventually be under 25%.

It is beyond the scope of this book to build a customized weight training program for you. So, please work with a personal trainer that understands the above principles. Don't be afraid to ask them about the above principles. Because you are hiring them . . . and they work for you!

ACTION STEP:

If you are older or injured, you can still lift weights. There is a functional system called, <u>Blood Flow Restriction Training</u>, it works by limiting blood flow to the muscle. Which allows for more satellite and stem cells to build and grow muscle. Without having to lift heavy weights.

That's weight training so, **What about cardio training?**

To do cardio correctly in our opinions you *do not have to do* cardio more than 3 times a week. You can do a lite walk around the block every night if you like . . . but we are talking about actual cardio training.

For example, riding a stationary bike or walking on a treadmill. For these types of exercise machines, we recommend the same confusion principle only adapted for cardio. So, say you were on the stationary bike, you would start off at a slow normal easy pace for 2 minutes. Just enough to get your blood flowing and then you will up the pace a more vigorous pace, just 70 to 75% of your fastest possible pace, and then stay there for 15 seconds. Then come back down to normal pace for 30 seconds. Then back up to a rigorous pace for 15 seconds - and back down to normal pace for 30 seconds. Do this back and forth routine for a total of 5 minutes. Then do a 2 minute warm down - breathing in thru your nose and slowly out, thru your mouth for 2 minutes.

For your next cardio training session you should vary the pace, or the time or the exercise machine for the confusion principle.

This is a type of <u>H.I.T. cardio</u>, aka cardio confusion, works because it taxes your nervous system which will then change your physiology and your body composition. . . <u>[video tutorial 25]</u>

To a more lean, less self conscience, more confident body image!

When you look good . . . You feel good!

Fun Fact:

We have all seen that person, who walks on the treadmill for 45 minutes 3 times a week. Religiously walking, sweating and still looking the exact same way . . . 3 months later! Because they never tax their nervous system (cardio confusion) their body composition never changes . .

*So.. . **Please, please, don't be that person!***

CHAPTER 5

THE INSULTHIN DIET AND GUT HEALTH

"If there's one thing to know about the human body; it's this: the human body has a ringmaster. This ringmaster controls your digestion, your immunity, your brain, your weight, your health and even your happiness. This ringmaster is the gut."
-Nancy Mure

The above quote really nails it, when it comes to describing our gut microbiome. First off, what is our gut microbiome?

Our gut is the home of trillions of microorganisms. There are over *1000 different kinds of microbes living in your digestive tract.* These bacteria, viruses and fungi, make up your gut microbiome. You can think of it like a very diverse garden. Your gut microbiome plays a key role in digesting the food you eat and absorbing and synthesizing nutrients from your food. Several factors influence your composition of gut microbiome. These factors include the microbiome we inherit from our mother's body, our diets, antibiotics and our lifestyle. Your microbiome, in turn, affects different aspects of your body like your metabolism, mood, and your immune system.

Believe it or not those bugs in our gut flora out number us by 900 trillion cells! And they have over 2 million genes, we have only 25 thousand. What does that mean?

1. There are more of them, then there are of us!

2. They are smarter than us: there is more communication from our gut to our brain than vice versa.

3. They can stop us from being anxious or depressed

4. They can prevent us from getting sick: over 70% of your immune system is in your gut microbiome.

5. They can help us or stop us from losing weight: there is direct communication, neurons, from your gut to your brain.

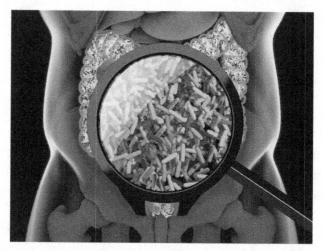

So just what is the link between your microbiome and your weight?

Recent research into the role of the gut microbiome in obesity has uncovered some fascinating links. One study exploring this link examined the gut bacteria in obese and lean mice and humans. They found that weight gain or loss was not connected to the amount or type of foods the mice or humans ate. When the researchers took the feces (poop) out of the fat mice and put it in the thin mice. The thin mice became fat. Conversely when they put the feces out of the thin mice and placed it in the fat mice, the fat mice became thin! Wow!

How's that for some exciting new news about weight loss?

This study showed that our gut microbiome plays an extremely important role in obesity. Several other studies show the effects of the gut microbiome on insulin resistance, inflammation, and fat deposition in the body. So it is in your best interest to keep your gut flora healthy and happy, so you can lose weight and keep it off for life!

There is only one cell layer between your gut lining and the rest of your body. It's called a tight junction and when they get loose (proteins uncouple) they create what's called leaky gut syndrome aka chronic disease . . .

Which ones? All of them!

Many metabolites (metabolomes), small particles we measure in your blood chemistry, are not human. What? You say . . .not human? Yes . . . that's right, they are up to ⅓ from your gut's bacteria. And they are *regulating your immune system, activating mitochondria, regulating DNA, balancing your brain chemistry (moods) and helping you fight diseases !*

So, let's take care . . special care of our gut microbiome by eating something to help them out, *fertilize our garden, with every meal.*

What could that be?

Good clean alkaline plant based fats. Such as avocado's, any green veggies, coconuts and all green salads with nice fresh pressed virgin olive oil and apple cider vinegar dressing.

Be sure and check out all the gut friendly salads in chapter 9.

Those above mentioned foods are a great help because they are pre-biotics.

Prebiotics are fibrous plant based foods that feed your good beneficial flora.in addition plants have fiber, phytonutrients, phytochemical, polyphenols.

We also recommend supplementing your microbiome with Ultra GI Max, every morning on an empty stomach. Because there are so many toxins in and around our environment, like pesticides, herbicides, insecticides and glycophosphates (round up), even if you are careful they can still get to you and disrupt your gut. Not to mention if you have to take medications like antacids, steroids, and anti inflammatories.

ACTION STEP:

You can test your own microbiome at home with the Thorne Gut Smart test kit.

Now we should mention that there are 3 types of probiotics:

1. **Dead probiotics** - these bugs feed on dead or decaying particles like, kimchi, kombucha, yogurt, kefir and sauerkraut. We DO NOT recommend these types of probiotics, because we are alive and vital, not dead and decaying.

2. **Standard probiotics** - these are the kind you find in the health food stores. They grow it in rich, organic non-GMO soil with enough sun, air, water and time for them to be alive and vital. These are much better than the dead probiotics (fermented).

3. **Elevated probiotics** - these are found on fruits, vegetables and lettuce (spinach, kale, etc.). If they are not washed and certified regenerative organic, there will be a whitish coating on them (sometimes it's microscopic). Those are probiotics from the sun . . . hence the name elevated probiotics. These types are the best to consume.

Dr. Tang, a researcher at the university of Connecticut, found out something amazing with plants and our microbiome. Plants RNA can go inside our gut bacteria (microsomes > exosomes) and *change their gene expression.* Which means it will do 3 things for you:

1. Change the metabolic rate of your flora. Which means they can raise your BMR and get you burning fat . . .faster.

2. Produce more of your neurotransmitters, like serotonin (happy hormone), dopamine (feel good hormone), oxytocin (I am in love hormone)

3. Help heal the lining of your intestines.(leaky gut syndrome)

These are super important reasons why we made the InsulThin **"plant rich"** diet. And why we say, make sure you include a gut healthy green salad or green veggie at every meal . . . and don't forget the Kerry butter!

The American Gut Project surveyed over 11,000 people and found that the **"the number one predictor of a healthy microbiome was the variety of plant foods consumed in one's diet"** . . . . **Hello? Are you'all listening?**

One of the most common gut imbalances that we see, in the clinic, is a Candida yeast, overgrowth. Brought on by our high carb / low fat diets, which of course make an abundance of sugar. And **Candida loves sugar!** And antibiotics, as any woman knows, who has taken antibiotics and gotten a yeast infection. Men have them as well, they are just not as visible.

We place our patients on our candida cleanse before we start them on the plant rich, InsulThin diet plan.

So, it should be clear to you that the critters inside your microbiome regulate several vital functions of your mind and body. In addition, any alterations in your gut microbiota have significant effects on your weight, your health and your well-being.

ACTION STEP:

Knowing your transient time is critical for your microbiome' health. Transient time is simply the time a food travels from your mouth to the toilet. How can you test it? Just eat a moderate helping of beets or corn (this is just for testing purposes and not part of diet). Then time how long it is until you see purple (beets) or the kernels of corn. It should take between 12 to 24 hours. If it's less than 12, food is going through you too fast. Try our Probiotics.

If that does not work, you need to see a Naturopath, Functional Medicine Doctor, Holistic Chiropractor. If it takes longer than 24 hours, you are constipated. Try a natural colon cleanse like Our Intestinal Cleanse.

If that does not work, . .. see an informed Health Care Specialist.

A couple of helpful hints, when you eat, make sure you chew your food until it's liquid (or darn close). Because your saliva has enzymes that help break down your food. Second, don't drink with your meal, *always drink before* or 1 hour after a meal. *Reason is you dilute your hydrochloric acid (HCL).* which causes you to not digest your food completely (dysbiosis).

And you also create something called, mucoid plaque. Mucoid plaque is like tooth plaque, it creates problems for you by interfering with your food absorption.

Interesting Fact

As you probably know, plants breathe carbon dioxide (CO_2) for life and expel oxygen (O_2) which of course is vital for our life. Isn't it very interesting that when you are in ketosis, 84% of your fat leaves through your exhalation as carbon dioxide (CO_2). Significance?

We give plants life, carbon dioxide CO_2, and they in turn give us life, oxygen (O_2).

Being on the InsulThin Diet plan is a beautiful cycle between us and our critically important cousins . . . life giving plants!

ACTION STEP:

Trying to lose weight with chest breathing is like trying to go when the light is green, with one foot on the gas and the other foot on the brake.

DEMO

Put 1 hand on your chest and the other on your stomach.

Breathe *into* your belly. Belly breathing takes in more oxygen than chest breathing. Belly breathing also activates your vagus nerve, which puts you into rest, digest and repair mode (parasympathetic).

1 More Interesting Fact

This relates to just how close we are related to plants. If you were to take the magnesium out of plants and exchange it with the "heme" in our hemoglobin. Then we would have cytoplasm, plant blood. And the plants would have plasma, human blood. *How is that for a close relationship?*

And this might be a good time to remind everyone that sunshine is necessary for both plants (obviously) and humans. Our skin is like a solar panel that picks up photons from the sun and charges our bodies and our brains. The tissue that made your brain (ectoderm) is the same tissue that made your skin (ectoderm). So don't be afraid of the sun . . . get out in the early morning hours, 8am to 11am. Or late afternoon, 5pm to 7 pm.

And charge up your brain!

In addition, just like plants are grounded to the earth.

We should be grounded to the earth as well! There are lots of reasons that go beyond the scope of this book . .

but a great resource is a book titled. . . . Earthing.

ACTION STEP:

Since rubber is on the bottom of most of our shoes. And rubber insulates us from the earth, we can go to Amazon and pick up these little straps (Earthling 3.0). They reconnect us, ground us, back to our life giving planet . . earth.

Corollary ACTION STEP

Your mouth has a very diverse microbiome and is different from your gut microbiome. Yet and still, it provides very important roles in digestion and nitric oxide production (NO). Nitric oxide is super important in your brain, heart and sexual function (Mr. Happy gets and stays happier- if you know what we mean). So we recommend Revitin toothpaste, it's made by Dentists. It will help gingivitis, halitosis (bad breath) and protect and build the bacteria that make your nitric oxide.

One Last Super Important Fact

Did you ever wonder . . . where do these super smart, super strong microbes get their energy to help us from?

Well as it turns out, they get their energy from fatty acids, not sugar (glucose), that make butyrate. That should sound familiar?

Because we on the InsulThin diet take fatty acids and make beta hydroxy - butyrate. And yes they are two different sides of the same coin.

Significance, your microbiome knows what the best fuel source is and

it's not . . . . sugar / insulin!

It's good healthy fats / ketones . . . because they have had *thousands of years* to perfect it!

So, your energy requirements are in good company, when you are on the InsulThin diet plan! [Video Tutorial 26]

CHAPTER 6

A DAY IN THE LIFE OF
"FAT ADAPTED" PERSON

"Yesterday was history, tomorrow is a mystery and today is a gift . . .
that's why it's called the present!"
Master Oogway

Ok, this is going to be fun . . . This is Dr. Grego speaking and this is a typical day in my fat adapted InsulThin life. A couple of things right from the start, you might have noticed that I said "fat adapted" and not "keto" so what is the difference?

Fat adapted is the next level of any type of keto, it means that I have graduated from just having ketones in my body to having my brain use primarily ketones for fuel. The difference being that if I urinated on a ketone strip it would not turn purple or pink. Because that type of ketone, aceto-acetate, will be all used up (no color change on ketone strip) when I reach true fat adaptation. Meaning I became more efficient at using ketones for fuel and my brain changed from primarily glucose to ketones for energy. (everyone doing the InsulThin Diet is fat adapted)

I know what some of you are thinking, "you can't use primarily ketones in the brain, we need at least 130 grams of carbs and glucose for our brains to function correctly!"

That's a great big . . . . Negative! This is a study by Dr. George Cayhill . . .

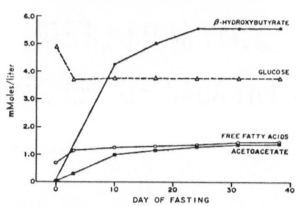

BLOOD GLUCOSE, FREE FATTY ACIDS
AND KETONE BODY LEVELS DURING FAST

FIG. 2. Circulating concentrations of βOHB, glucose, free fatty acids and acetoacetate in obese but otherwise normal man fasting for 40 days (9).

This study shows conclusively that even when fasting blood sugar went down to around *20mg/dl (which would normally mean coma and certain death),* they then injected 20 IU of insulin. With insulin injected into the subjects at that low level, ***no one passed out, went into a coma, or had any symptoms of low blood sugar (hypoglycemia).*** "Wow" . . . but how can that be?

That's the power of ketones and a fat adapted brain! And this study shows just how protective and supportive and superior, ketones are over glucose/insulin, for you and your brain!

Now, if I wished to test my ketone levels I would use a precision xtra meter to see if I was over 1 mM. However I use something much cheaper and more efficient, in my opinion, the **"taste test"**. This is where I take the end of my finger and wet it with my saliva. And then dip it in white sugar, and interestingly enough if I taste *"nothing or sheet rock dust"* . . .

I am fat adapted. [video tutorial 27]

If I taste sweet . . . I am not fat adapted.

Much simpler wouldn't you agree?

So, with that out of the way, the first thing I do when I wake up and get on my knees and say . . .

Good morning to God and to my son, Sean, who graduated (passed on) early at the age of 18.

Then while on my knees I stretch out and do DDP (Diamond Dallas Page) Yoga morning routine. It's available for free on YouTube. This only takes 2 minutes and is extremely helpful for flexibility in my spine and overall body. And it kept Mr. Page away from back surgery.

Then I do JAPA meditation. It is also available for free on YouTube just type in Wayne Dyer - Morning Ahh Guided Meditation for Manifesting Affirmations. This centers me and gets me focused and present for the day.

I only do this for 2 minutes as well.

Then I do a hot and cold shower to work out my cardio-vascular system. Arteries are muscles and hot water relaxes them and cold water contracts them. And what is anaerobic exercise? Contracting and relaxing muscles . . . that's what I do in the shower for my arteries (muscles) which helps my heart. [video tutorial 29]

Then I eat breakfast . . . ah . . no . . . just kidding! No I do not break - fast with breakfast, my eating window is 5 hours. It's from 1 pm to 6 pm. So I am in a fasted state for 18 hours a day, from my last meal at 6 pm all night and morning long until my first meal at 1 pm. Of course I drink alkalized water (Life Ionizer) all day long, with a pinch of Celtic sea salt in the water.

Usually I am so busy in the mornings I don't even think about or desire food. And no, I am never hungry in the mornings. So my first meal is a Beyond meat burger cooked in lots of Kerry butter with sriracha and Boar's head mustard. Along with lightly steamed asparagus dipped in butter. And a side kale and baby spinach salad topped with avocado and sliced almonds. Boy doesn't that sound delicious? But the reality is, most days I am too busy to cook all that. . . . so I open a jar of Dr. Bronner coconut oil and a jar of Santa Cruz peanut butter and a couple tablespoons of both. Which happens to be 100 grams of good healthy fat! And for my colon, I would just grab a handful of baby spinach or kale. And of course I chew until it's liquid and I never drink when I eat. Of course I say a quick prayer first, "God thank you for this food and bless it for the nourishment of my body . . Amen." Nothing like a little attitude of gratitude to open your life for blessings . . . Amen?

Then for dessert (LOL), I chew my vitamins, with a tablespoon of Dr. Bronner's coconut oil. Why chew vitamins? Because any absorption problems are circumvented . . . when chewing my vitamins they are absorbed through insalivation (sides of the cheek) and sublingually (under the tongue). A much more efficient and faster way to get vitamins into your system. Why chew with coconut oil? Coconut oil is a healthy fat of course, and acts as a liposomal delivery system. A liposomal delivery system is the fastest most effective way to get any vitamin or mineral into a human body. Because our cells have a double fat layer called phospho-lipid membranes.

And simply put when fat meets fat they mingle much better.

[video tutorial 30]

My vitamins I take on a daily basis are as follows:

Intestinal Cleanser - because everything we eat does not always go through us!

Probiotics - because our gut microbiome is the "ringmaster" of our body.

Thyroid/Adrenal - because we can't pick family members or our bosses! (they can cause adrenal stress-lol)

Vitamin D3 / K2 (liposomal) - because we don't get out in the sun enough. And we were on fat free diets. Vitamin D is made from cholesterol (fat)

Digestive Enzymes - because we cook and therefore kill enzymes in our foods.

Collagen Peptides - these keep your joints strong. And keep you looking younger because they hold elasticity in your connective tissues.

Mothers Earth Core + pH Balancer- because our soil is depleted of vitamins and minerals. In addition we are super acidic because of ultra processed foods. That's why we need regenerative farming.

*Fulvic acid - because it has all of the essential amino acids and vitamins and minerals that we need to be healthy. But fulvic acid is not in our produce. Because our farmers use fungicides and kill the fungus

(Phanerochaete chrysosporium) responsible for making fulvic acid. Which means there is no breaking down dead animal parts, leaves, rotten fruit, etc.

That would normally give us back the nutrients we need for our health. And fulvic also helps repair leaky-gut syndrome.

Yet another reason for regenerative farming!

*If my gut microbiome was in terrible shape or if I was immune challenged, I would enhance my probiotics with GI ProMAX GUT to supercharge my microbiota.

Rapid Ketosis - I drink 1 teaspoon right before bedtime. It drops me deeper into ketosis. It changes any white fat to brown fat.

Fun Fact:

"IF I WAS TRAPPED ON A DESERTED ISLAND . . . AND COULD ONLY TAKE 1 SUPPLEMENT IT WOULD BE . . . . FULVIC ACID!"

And a corollary with coconut oil, if you happen to have loose teeth, you can do oil pulling and tighten up those loose teeth. Just by pulling (sucking) the coconut oil back and forth between you lose teeth for 1 minute. Then satisfied and full I go through my day, saying to myself, *why is this such a beautiful day?* I say that to myself (self talk) so my reticular activating system (RAS) looks for things that are "beautiful".

You see our subconscious minds are programmed to only answer thoughts stated in the positive. For example, if you tell a child - "don't spill the milk" - what do they do? Spill the milk, because they like you do not hear the "don't" - their subconscious only hears -"spill the milk" . . . and now you know why they spilled the "milk".

So check your self talk and restate your language, in the positive, if you need to?

Then I go to work (practice) where I work out. We have weights and machines in the office, so I train before I see patients. I always do weight training first to burn off any extra glucose that I might have from the previous day's eating (hopefully not). And when I train with weights it's all about the time under tension principle for muscle density. Along with the muscle confusion principle, which is changing up the types of exercise and or the cadence of the movement and or the angle of the movement.

Reason is our nervous system is quick to adapt to any stressor (exercise) and then will not change our body composition (i.e. lean body muscle or fat %).

Then I do cardio, only 4 minutes of H.I.T. (high intensity training). Which I very (cardio confusion) the time, for example 10 seconds of high intensity and 20 seconds of normal intensity for 4 min. Then the next session 15 seconds of high intensity and 15 seconds of normal intensity for 4 min. Remembering again that our nervous systems are very quick to adapt and need to be challenged in a different way, every time we work out.

Or we will be that dreaded person who sweats and toils for 45 min. on the treadmill, 3 to 4 times a week. Doing cardio and yet, looks exactly the same 3 months later . . . sad.

Now as I go through my day, of course, *not everything is beautiful.* And I adjust to the *challenges (not problems)* by looking for lessons or the good in the undesirable people - places and things that *I created throughout the day.* Notice that I said I "created" as opposed to the things that "happened" to me, because I am choosing to make my circumstances, by saying that I "created" them. As opposed to saying, "I can't believe that happened to me!". Thereby becoming a victim of people-places and things.

We can either be a creator or a victim in our lives. [video tutorial 31]

And being a creator is much more fun!

Also people sometimes say "no" to my desires, so when I hear opposition, like when someone tells me an answer I don't want to hear. For example "no" I am sorry we can't do that for you. Instead of asking, "well why not?", which will get me a laundry list of all the reasons and rationale to support why it's "not" going to happen . . .so instead I ask,

"Ok, I understand it's not possible, and let me ask you a question, hypothetically, if it were possible for what I am asking to work, what would have to happen?"

and 9 times out of 10 they will tell me what I could do to make it happen, and if it's not unrealistic . . . I do it and get satisfaction! All because I trained myself to ask a better question.

If I snack at all during the day, I snack on raw almonds (with celtic sea salt), they are full of good fat and also happen to be the most alkaline nut on the planet.

I also ran out to my Chiropractor, to get checked, to see if I need a "tune-up"?

No I don't have any back pain and no I have not been in an auto accident (Thank God) . . . I, like most of my patients, find that just like a car . . . we run better when tuned-up! You might consider it for yourself, as well?

What I drink is not as important as when I drink.

And **I always drink before I eat, never when I eat.**

Because if I drink when I eat, I will dilute my hydrochloric acid. Hydrochloric acid is my stomach acid and it's supposed to be 1.5 to 2.0 pH. It is very acidic, so it can digest my food properly. If I drink anything above 2.0 pH (which is everything) then I will dilute my stomach acid, not digest my food properly, and create mucoid plaque. Mucoid plaque is just like tooth plaque in that it stains your intestines and interrupts proper absorption from our bowels.

Who says that? Well only the world's foremost authority on bowel function, Dr. Hiromi Shinyna. Dr. Shinya is the creator of the colonoscopy machine. He has personally performed over 350k colonoscopies. **He boasts a 0% recidivism (recurrence) rate for colon cancer.** For those you adopt his eating and drinking plan.

And routinely advises patients not to drink when they eat (mucoid plaque) and use alkalized water (Life Ionizer) after they eat. That said, I never drink when I eat, always 5 minutes before my meal. And one hour after my meals.

Then for dinner I will have blackened salmon (wild caught), make sure it's not Atlantic salmon, because salmon don't swim in the Atlantic. That's another name for pond raised salmon. So, I will have the wild caught salmon blackened in a cast iron skillet with lots of Kerry butter and Chef Paul's blackened seasoning. With a side of steamed brussel sprouts seasoned with celtic sea salt and of course lots of Kerry butter. And a side mixed greens salad topped with baked coconut pieces, Chao cheese and raw sunflower seeds. The dressing is extra virgin olive oil (fresh pressed) and apple cider vinegar with a few drops of liquid stevia.

I will always take a digestive enzyme because any time I cook food, *I kill the enzymes in that food.* So, we should help out our digestion with a digestive enzyme . . . make sense? If I have dessert it will be a choice between: Rebel chocolate ice cream is absolutely delicious with only 5 net carbs. Or a ChocZero peanut butter cups very tasty with only monk fruit sugar. Then one hour later, I will take 2 Rapid Ketosis and take digestive enzyme since I cooked some of the food. Remember, we kill the enzymes when we cook our food. And I feel compelled to share with you on a deeper level, why you and I have to take digestive enzymes . . . but don't we have them already? Short answer is Negative. . . because you and I don't eat 80% raw food and 20% cooked food. You and I eat more like the opposite, 20% raw and 80% cooked. And that means we don't replenish our enzyme population. Ergo - vis-a-vis - you and I need to take enzymes to fully break down our foods and get all the good nutrition into our cells.

Make sense?

Before I retire, I will turn off my Wi-Fi/router (EMF's) and turn off my phone and computer. Looking at either of those two things will interrupt my sleep. Because non-native blue light disrupts circadian rhythms and deep sleep. And then I ask myself a question,

"What is one thing that I can be grateful for today?"

and then I feel better about my day and my life. I then make sure I am breathing from my belly. Because if my chest moves first when I take a deep breath, then I am in sympathetic mode (fight or flight) and it will be hard for me to go to sleep.

If I take 3 big breaths in thru the nose, hold it for 3-5 seconds, then out. I breathe from my belly, because then I will reset my vagus nerve and be in parasympathetic mode (rest and repair). If I still have a hard time getting to sleep,

I will go to Brain Tap and find a program [video tutorial 32]

Called "delta" and listen until I fall asleep.

At which point I will go to sleep. Binaural beats are simply offsetting frequencies that you listen to and then your brain entrains (comes together) with one desired frequency. In the case of delta (deep sleep) that frequency is between 1 to 4 hrtz.

Fun Fact:

I brush my teeth with Revitin toothpaste. Because regular toothpaste has a "warning label" on the back of them, that reads: "if more toothpaste used for brushing is accidently swallowed, call the Poison Control Center right away!". Why would it say that? Because the fluoride used in your toothpaste is the *active ingredient in rat poison.*

ACTION STEP:

Use Revitin toothpaste because Revitin was made by Dentists to help support your mouth's unique microbiome. It also helps gingivitis and halitosis (bad breath).

Some of you might be thinking? What are his macros? What are his micro's? I know there's too much sugar in there somewhere? Those meals and desserts aren't perfect !? To which I answer . . . .

Stop it! Stop it! . . . Stop over *analy*zing!

In my opinion - Life and being Keto are less rules and more about being . . . being happy, and not setting up so many rules. The more rules you have in life . . . the harder it is and the more miserable it is! We are not purists . . . just pragmatists . . . trying to live life without too much of what I call the double DD's - Disease and Disaster! Who's with me? I think Shakespeare said it best when he said. . .

"Tragedies in life are inevitable, but misery is a choice." - Shakespeare

CHAPTER 7

5 QUESTIONS YOU MUST ASK BEFORE STARTING INSULTHIN DIET

"Many people want to live right. Their concern with right living makes them focus on themselves and the things they struggle with. But it is right believing, that produces right living."
Pastor Joseph Prince

1st Question You Must Ask Yourself:

What's most important to me in my life?
What has to happen in order for me to feel that?

If you honestly and openly ask and answer these 2 questions, they will give you your number one core *value* in your life.

Your core value is the most significant thing in your life is something you should know because...

"... if you want to be successful and live a happy and fulfilled life. Then you must know what your core value is ... and ...

you must experience it on a daily basis!"
-Tony Robbins

Then you can use the answer to motivate you to do the InsulThin LifeStyle, which will allow you . . . to become more vibrant and be better able to achieve that which you truly desire.

For example, if you answered, *"my children are the most important to me in my life."*

And in order for me to feel them, *"I must be active and play with them."*

Then you will need all the energy, strength, and vibrancy to be able to do that on a daily basis. So being on the InsulThin Diet will give you that opportunity to do what's most important to you . . .

Does that make sense?

2nd Question:
Is to find out your limiting beliefs.

To do this you must close your eyes and ask yourself this question . . .

If I could know what was holding me back from starting and enjoying the InsulThin Lifestyle, it would be?

With this question you will discover your limiting belief, that's keeping you from doing this appealing lifestyle. Please ask it sincerely and the first thought that comes up will be the correct reason why or what's potentially holding you back from doing the InsulThin LifeStyle . . .

The answer to replacing your limiting belief(s) are two fold:

1 You must attach negative or painful associations to your limiting beliefs

Example: "I can't give up carbs!" -

BUT *they are just sugar in disguise and sugar destroys my*

body and makes me feel achy and tired then I'll miss playing with my children!

2 Second part of destroying limiting beliefs is to reframe your limiting statement.

Example: "I can't give up carbs!" - BECOMES -

"Why is giving up carbs so easy for me?

That is not just semantics - This is real science based on your subconscious mind and something called the RAS (reticular activating system).

RAS is a little beyond the scope of this book, so if you want to learn more I have linked a definition for it. Link is here, also Dr. Joe Dispenza does a great job on showing you how to focus your mind to get what you want . . . link here.

3rd Question:

Do I have a resource, a guide, someone I can call or talk to? If I have any questions or challenges while getting into this new LifeStyle?

If you answered no ... Stop right now and find someone!

Even Michael Jordan had a Coach!

Be it an informed medical doctor, chiropractor, naturopath or holistic doctor or certified health coach.

You don't have to physically go there, but you can Skype them, Video chat, or FaceTime them, but you must have a good caring professional who understands the ins and outs of the InsulThin LifeStyle.

You may consider reaching out to us at:

Free Consultation/Webinar

Dr. Grego on

Dr. Grego Keto Doc on

Or

Dr. Grego Keto Doc on

4th Question:

*Do I have the best ketone supplement to
help me get in and stay in Keto?*

**Remember you can try and you may even succeed in getting into
Keto. But it is soooo much easier, in these authors' opinion, to use
a proper Ketone Supplement.**

Here is the best one because it has fat emulsifiers to break up your own
fat.

1. Extra Strength Rapid Ketosis

It is imperative that your ketone supplement has fat emulsifiers, so you
can start making your own ketones. And increase the Keto effect more
intensely.

*Because otherwise you will potentially shut down your own ketone
factory (negative feedback loop) by continuously giving yourself
ketones from the outside.. . . make sense?*

And that is never a good thing and NOT something you want to do. . .
period.

The reason why we bring this important point up is because there is only 1 ketone supplement available, as of this writing, is that has fat emulsifiers in it . . . . can you guess which one?

Rapid Ketosis of course!

Also exogenous ketones **help turn ugly harmful white fat into good metabolically active brown fat.**

They also can help shrink . . .a fatty liver!

5th Question:

Do I want to hug fat? . . . .or

Do I want to fight fat?

This really gets to the heart of the matter.

Sometimes we just over think things.

We make things more complicated than they need to be.

Weight loss just might be one of those things.

Let's see if we can clear the air here . . . with regards to you simply losing weight.

In this column is the Pro's

Weight Loss w/ The InsulThin Diet:

1. It increases fat burning (ketosis)

2. It increases your BMR (nervous system ramps up)

3. It increases energy (fat = 9 kCal/gram vs carbs= 4 kCal/gram)

4. It increases satiety (you get fuller faster- wont overeat)

5. It increase brown fat (metabolically active good fat)

6. It protects valuable muscle (when you lose 10 lbs. it's all fat)

7. It increases sex drive (all your sex hormones are made from fat)

8. Decreases fatty liver

In this column are the Con's

For Weight Loss with Protein / Low Calorie / Low Fat diets:

Weight Watchers - Jenny Craig - Nutrisystem - Mediterranean diet - Atkins - Paleo - Carnivore -

Your uniformed doctors' advice - your dietician's advice - your nutritionist advise - your personal trainers advice - the biggest losers diet - DASH diet - Volumetrics diet - Mayo Clinic Diet - Ornish diet - Nordic diet - MIND diet - TLC diet -your next door neighbors advice - your friends advice - your own advice

1. It stops fat burning (lipolysis) & makes fat (De novo lipogenesis)

2. It decreases BMR (down regulates nervous system)

3. It decreases your energy (Krebs cycle: carbs 36 ATP - Ketones 146 ATP)

4. It increases your hunger pains (Ghrelin increases- your I am hungry hormone)

5. It increases white fat (bad visceral fat)

6. It burns valuable muscle (when you lose 10lbs - 5 = fat 5 = muscle)

7. It decreases your sex drive (low calorie lowers testosterone)

When you compare The InsulThin Diet to every other diet out there . .

it becomes . . Painfully obvious, as the nose on your face . . .

as to which way you should go . . . isn't that . . so?

Common Sense Fact:

What is the . . .best way . . to get a vitamin . . or any nutrient . .

Into . . .our bodies?

With a . . . "Liposomal" (fat) delivery system . . . .which is. . . .

wait for it. . . .

FAT!

Why is that. . . You ask?

Simple . . . . Everyone of your cells . . .has not 1 . . but 2 layers . . .

Of . . . . .Fat . . .called. . . Phospho-lipid (fat) Membranes . . . .

And . . .Fat . . .mingles better . . . with Fat . . . Period.

CHAPTER 8

SUMMARIZING THE BOOK

"If you want to be happy, practice compassion. If you want others to be happy . . Practice . . . compassion."
-Dali Lama

How to do The InsulThin Diet in 7 Easy Steps

"Always ask, will what I am about to eat,
Protect my Brain + Feed my Gut?"

1 Stop buying/putting ultra processed high carb low fat foods in your body

2 Start **Focusing on Insulin** - 15% spike or less -

by eating more good healthy fats/fiber caps

Use **Insulin Calculator** (to control insulin spikes 15% or <)

    a. Look at InsulThin food / Grocery lists / InsulThin Recipes

    b. Drink before meal - never during

3 Eat a Salad or a green veggie (w/ fiber cap) with every meal.

a. Chew until liquid

b. eat ½ meal then text friend - (Leptin)

c. Your plate should look 75% green veggies 25% protein w/ a bowl of melted butter

3 Pick a tighter Eating Window (EW) 4 to 6 hours. Or OMAD.

a. Start Rapid Ketosis > 2 capsules before every meal + at night before bed.

4 Use melted Butter - Fresh Olive Oil - Coconut Oil every day.

5 Do the "taste test" check if sugar tastes like "nothing or sheet rock dust"

a. If sugar still tastes sweet = not fat-adapted . . . yet.

b. Get with a Healthcare Professional = consider our Coaches

6 Start weight training and cardio

a. Weight training = time under tension + muscle confusion principles

b. Cardio = cardio confusion principles + breathe: nose into belly

7 Look in a full length mirror and **"if"** you like what you see . . .

Congrats!

Share the InsulThin Diet, with someone you know love or care

about!

A quick note when you go grocery shopping . . . as a general rule, you should:

Buy groceries that are located around the outside edges of the store. Because they contain mostly whole foods and not ultra processed foods. And be very careful, read the labels, on the foods located in the center of the grocery stores. Make sure they come from a regenerative source.

We believe Dr. Jason Fung might have said it best when he said . . .

"Insulin levels are what drives everything, it drives metabolic disease (diabetes, Alzheimer's, high blood pressure, obesity) it drives heart disease, it drives strokes, it drives cancer!"

Dr. Jason Fung

We say . . . ."Don't let insulin drive you to the hospital or an early grave . .

Instead drive without insulin to a much happier and healthier life . . ." With the InsulThin Diet Plan!

Remember when you build your health . . . .

You put money in the bank, because you are not spending it on medications or hospitals!

"Best way to build Wealth is to build Health!"

Finally, good healthy fats are natural and safe for you to eat. They will help you lose weight and feel great, they will help you live longer and feel better about yourself. Your understanding of fats (not trans fats) has been tainted by the food industry's propaganda.

Which is bent on profit over health.

Please don't let their lies sway you

God started you burning fat - the food industry made you fat, with a plethora of tempting ultra processed foods. Which are incredibly overused in your daily food and drink choices. They can and do make health problems that destroy your health. Because of your insulin response to ultra processed foods, which make you sick and obese. Which ultimately makes you die - in - pieces. A tortuous death at best. So lighten up (pun intended) and embrace good healthy fats and the InsulThin Lifestyle . . .

You will be glad you did! [video tutorial 34]

With that said, we will say . . . that's all for now . . .

Live your life - Out loud and Fat Adapted!

Dr. Mike Grego   Kevin Grego   Tonda Parham

PS

As of the writing of this book my brother, Kevin, has just uncovered a Harvard trained scientist (David Sinclair) who says he has reversed aging in animal models (mice). He says in a nutshell

The secrets to humans living forever are:

1. Intermittent fasting - ideally only 1 meal a day (OMAD)

2. Cold/Hot showers - staying a little colder or hotter than you like through the day

3. Eating no animal proteins

Does this sound familiar?

A lot like the plant rich based InsulThin diet?

You can watch the video here.

CHAPTER 9

INSULTHIN DIET DELICIOUS RECIPES AND DRINKS

"The doctor of the future will give no medicine, but will interest his patient in the care of the human frame, in diet and in the cause and prevention of disease."
T .Edison

Delicious InsulThin Recipes

*All recipes have a percentage next to them - this is the % spike

of Insulin which should be 15% or less

Breakfast / Smoothies

InsulThin Coffee 4%

(if you have adrenal fatigue do not drink coffee)

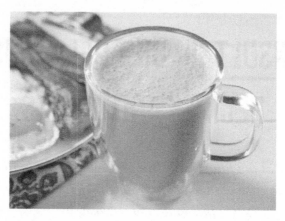

"Click <u>Underlined Colored Word</u> ingredients to buy them!"

Ingredients

1 tbsp. Kerry butter
1 tbsp. Coconut oil
5 drops of liquid Stevia/Monk fruit
A pinch of Celtic sea salt
Your favorite brand organic coffee

Instructions

1. Brew your favorite organic coffee and pour into a french press.
2. Then pour coffee out of the press into the blender.
3. Place butter, coconut oil, stevia/monk fruit and salt into a blender.
4. Blend and pour into your favorite coffee mug.
5. Enjoy!

Pistachio 10% Green Smoothie

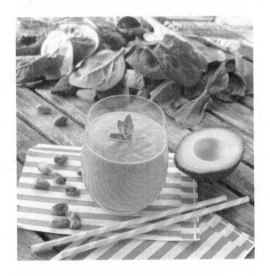

"Click <u>Underlined Colored Word</u> ingredients to buy them!"

Ingredients

$^1/_2$ average avocado (100 g/ 3.5 oz)
$^1/_4$ cup <u>Coconut milk</u> *or* heavy whipping cream
$^1/_4$ cup fresh spinach
1 medium <u>avocado</u>
fresh mint *or* mint extract to taste
$^1/_4$ cup <u>Solutions 4 Vanilla Shake</u>
2 tbsp. <u>Pistachio nuts</u> (unsalted) (20 g/ 0.7 oz)
1 tsp <u>Sweet drops vanilla extract</u>
3-6 drops <u>liquid Stevia extract</u> *or* <u>Monk fruit powder</u>
$^1/_2$ <u>Life Ionizer</u> alkalized water/ Evian and optionally ice cubes

Instructions

1. Wash the mint and spinach, halve and peel the avocado and blend until smooth with the rest of the ingredients.
2. Serve immediately.

Chocolate Peanut Butter Smoothie 14% (with 2 fiber caps)

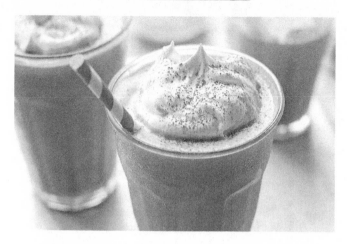

"Click Underlined Colored Word ingredients to buy them!"

Click underlined ingredients to buy them!

Ingredients

1/4 cup Santa Cruz creamy or crunchy peanut butter
3 tbsp. Cocoa powder
1 cup Heavy cream (or coconut cream for dairy-free or vegan)
1 1/2 cup Unsweetened almond milk (regular or vanilla)
6 tbsp. Monk fruit powder or liquid Stevia (to taste)
1/8 tsp Celtic sea salt
1 Avocado
!/2 cup of ice
Sliced almonds

Instructions

1. Combine all ingredients in a blender.
2. Puree until smooth. Adjust sweetener to taste if desired.
3. Add heavy whipping cream on top w/ sliced almonds

Oreo Shake 11%

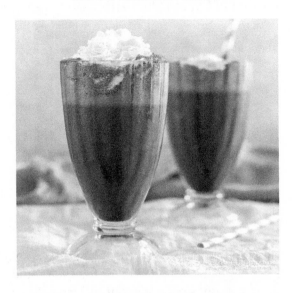

"Click <u>Underlined Colored Word</u> ingredients to buy them!"

Ingredients

1 ¹/₂ cups unsweetened almond milk, (12 fl oz)
¹/₄ cup heavy whipping cream (2 fl oz)
4 large eggs
1 medium avocado
4 tbsp. roasted Almond butter (2.3 oz)
3 tbsp. powdered Monk Fruit or Stevia (30 g/ 1.1 oz)
3 tbsp. Cacao powder (16 g/ 0.6 oz)
¹/₄ tsp sweet drops vanilla
¹/₂ cup whipped cream for topping (120 ml/ 4 fl oz)

Instructions

1. Pour the almond milk in an ice tray and freeze. You can skip this step if you don't want your shake frozen or use ice cubes instead.
2. Place the frozen almond milk and cream in a blender.
3. Add the eggs
4. Add the almond butter, sweetener, cacao powder and vanilla.
5. Process until smooth and creamy.
6. Pour into serving glasses
7. Top with whipped cream just before serving.

Granola Cereal 12% (with 2 fiber caps)

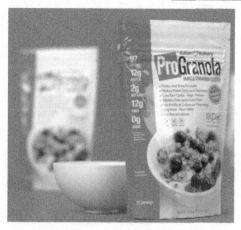

That's right this delicious vanilla breakfast cereal - peanut butter cereal - chocolate cereal - with all the flavor and . . .
It will not knock you out of ketosis!

Chorizo Omelets 12% (with 2 fiber caps)

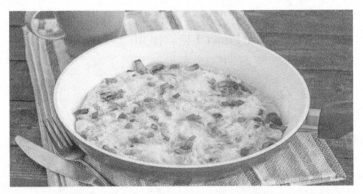

"Click Underlined Colored Word ingredients to buy them!"

Ingredients

2 large eggs
1/4 Cup Spinach, Chopped
2 Tablespoons White Onion
2 tablespoons Heavy Whipping Cream
2 Ounces of Chorizo
1/4 Cup Cheddar Cheese, Shredded
Celtic sea Salt & Pepper to Taste

Toppings

1 Tbsp. Sour Cream
1/8 cup of diced avocado
1 Slice of Bacon, Crumbled

Instructions

1. Cook Chorizo According to Package Instructions
2. In a medium bowl, whisk eggs, spinach, heavy whipping cream, and onion.
3. Pour mixture into non-stick skillet at low to medium heat
4. Flip omelet when firm enough. Cover omelet briefly with lid if not firming up
5. Sprinkle Cheese on other side and cook evenly
6. Remove from heat and place on plate
7. Add Chorizo to omelet and roll egg

8. Top with Sour Cream, Diced Avocado, Bacon and more Chorizo

InsulThin Toast 14% (with 2 fiber caps)

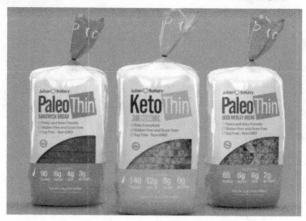

Now you can have your eggs with toast . . . .
This is Julian bakery's InsulThin Bread . . .make sure you add the butter!

Eggs Bacon and Avocado Breakfast 9%
(w 1 fiber cap)

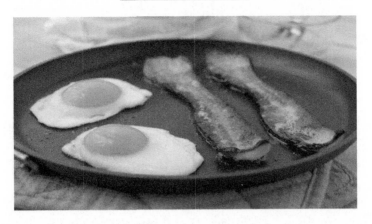

"Click Underlined Colored Word ingredients to buy them!"

Ingredients

2 slices bacon
2 eggs
1 tbsp. freshed pressed Olive Oil
Celtic sea salt and pepper
1 avocado diced
1 green onion

Instructions

1. Cook bacon to preferred crispiness and set aside.
2. Fry eggs in Kerry butter.
3. In a medium skillet, melt butter over medium-low heat.
4. Add eggs and cook until scrambled and done.
5. Top with green onion, bacon, and set avocado off to the side.
6. Place on plate and enjoy!

Cinnamon Roll Waffles 12%
(with 2 fiber caps)

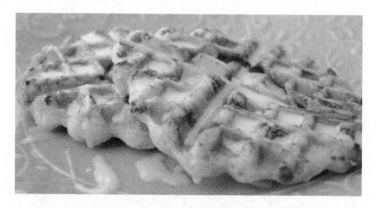

"Click Underlined Colored Word ingredients to buy them!"

Ingredients

Waffle Batter Ingredients

4 eggs
4 oz true whip topping
1 cup keto pancake mix
1 tsp sweet drops vanilla
1 tsp baking powder
1/3 cup Monk fruit powder

Cinnamon Swirl Ingredients

2 tbsp. melted Kerry butter
2 tbsp. liquid stevia
2 tbsp. Cinnamon

Icing Ingredients

4 oz True Whip Topping

Instructions

1. Put the cream cheese and process until smooth. Add the other ingredients and pulse until they are thoroughly incorporated.
2. Stir together the ingredients for the cinnamon swirl.

3. Spray your waffle iron with cooking spray. Spoon on the batter and drizzle on some of the cinnamon swirl. Swirl it in gently with a toothpick, knife, or spoon.
4. Cook until golden brown. Remove carefully. Repeat until all the batter is used up.
5. While the waffles are cooking stir together icing ingredients and set aside. Divide the icing between the waffles and serve

Note:
This makes 4 Belgian Waffles.

InsulThin Stuffed Avocado 10%

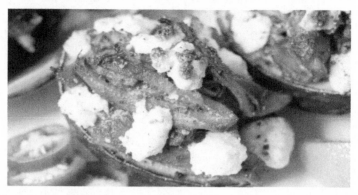

"Click <u>Underlined Colored Word</u> ingredients to buy them!"

Ingredients

3 slices of <u>bacon</u>
1 <u>avocado</u>
4 cherry tomatoes
¼ tsp <u>lime juice</u>
Pinch of <u>garlic</u>
<u>Celtic sea salt</u> / pepper to taste

Instructions

1. Cook the bacon.
2. Prep the avocados. Once you slice the avocados in half, remove the pit. Scoop half of the flesh out of each avocado half and transfer to a bowl.
3. Mix the filling. Mash the avocado and then stir in grape tomatoes, lettuce, lime juice, garlic powder, celtic sea salt, and black pepper. Gently mix in the chopped bacon.
4. Fill the avocados. Add the stuffing back into the avocado halves. ENJOY!

InsulThin Taco Breakfast Skillet 8% (with 2 fiber caps)

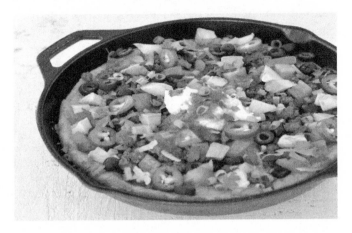

"Click Underlined Colored Word ingredients to buy them!"

Ingredients

1 pound ground beef or Beyond meat ground meat
4 tablespoons Taco Seasoning
2/3 cup water Life Ionizer or Evian
10 large eggs
1 1/2 cups shredded sharp cheddar cheese
1/4 cup heavy cream
1 roma tomato, diced
1 medium avocado, peeled, pitted and cubed
1/4 cup sliced black olives
2 green onions, sliced
1/4 cup sour cream
1/4 cup salsa
1 jalapeno, sliced (optional)
2 tablespoons cilantro
2 tbsp. Fresh Pressed Olive Oil

Instructions

1. Brown the ground meat in a large skillet with Olive Oil over medium-high heat. Drain the excess fat.
2. To the skillet, stir in the taco seasoning and water. Reduce the heat to low and let simmer until the sauce has thickened

and coats the meat. About 5 minutes. Remove half of the seasoned beef from the skillet and set aside.

3. Crack the eggs into a large mixing bowl and whisk. Add 1 cup of the cheddar cheese, and the heavy cream to the eggs and whisk to combine.

4. Preheat the oven to 375°F.

5. Pour the egg mixture over top of the meat retained in the skillet and stir to mix the meat into the eggs. Bake for 30 minutes, or until the egg bake is cooked all the way through and fluffy.

6. Top with remaining ground beef, the remaining ½ cup of cheddar cheese, tomato, avocado, olives, green onion, sour cream, and salsa.

7. Garnish with jalapeno and cilantro, if using.

InsulThin Bacon Stuffed Peppers 12%
<u>(1 fiber caps)</u>

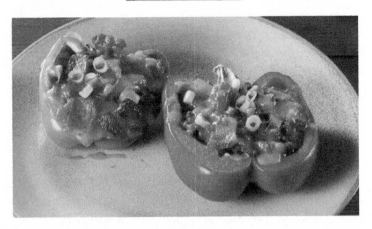

"Click <u>Underlined Colored Word</u> ingredients to buy them!"

Ingredients

1 Large Bell Pepper Any color
3 Eggs
3 Strips of <u>Bacon</u>
4 Small Mushrooms
1 cup Uncooked Spinach
1/2 cup Shredded <u>Cheddar Cheese</u>
2 - 3 Tbsp. <u>Fresh Pressed Olive Oil</u>

Instructions

1. Start by preheating your oven to 350 degrees and warming up the olive oil in a frying pan on your stovetop using medium heat.
2. While the pan is warming you can chop your mushrooms and your bacon to your desired size.
3. Place your bacon and mushrooms into the frying pan and cook on the stovetop until the bacon has started to crisp. While the bacon and mushrooms are cooking, use a bowl to whisk your eggs, but don't add them to the pan just yet.
4. we have to wait until the bacon has started to crisp.
5. At this time, measure out your spinach and favorite cheese. I recommend cheddar, but hey, you do you!

6. Once the bacon has started to crisp it is now time to add your eggs to the frying pan. I put the eggs and spinach in at the same time and let everything mix together, just like a scramble.

7. While that is cooking cut the top off your bell pepper and then place the pepper on its side. Slice the pepper in half horizontally, starting from the opened top all the way to the bottom and place in a casserole dish or on a baking sheet.

8. Now that your scramble is cooked to your liking, you're now ready to stuff the peppers. Once stuffed, sprinkle your cheese on top.

9. Place your peppers in the oven and let them bake for approximately 10 minutes at 350 degrees. This will allow the cheese to melt and the peppers will soften, but will still remain just firm and crunchy enough that you can pick them up to eat.

Chocolate Chip Pancakes 12%
(with 2 fiber caps)

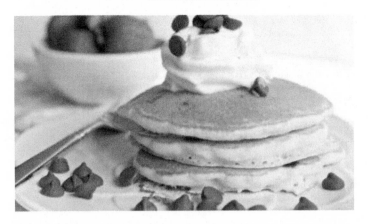

"Click Underlined Colored Word ingredients to buy them!"

Ingredients

2/3 cup Birch Benders Keto Pancake & Waffle Mix
1/2 cup Life Ionizer or Evian water
2 tbsp. Choczero chocolate chips
½ cup of heavy whipping cream
1 - 2 Tbsp. of Fresh Pressed Olive Oil

Instructions

1. Mix Birch Benders keto pancake mix with water in a bowl.
2. Heat up olive oil in a skillet over medium heat.
3. Add a fourth of the batter to the skillet. Let the batter cook on one side for 2-3 minutes and then flip.
4. Repeat with remainder of the pancake batter.
5. Divide the pancakes between two plates.
6. Top with heavy whipping cream and choczero chips.

Waffle Breakfast Sandwich 12%
(with 2 fiber caps)

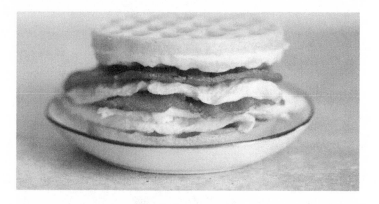

"Click <u>Underlined Colored Word</u> ingredients to buy them!"

Ingredients

3/4 cup Birch Benders Keto Pancake & Waffle Mix
1/2 cup Life Ionizer or Evian water
2 eggs
3 slices bacon
2 slices cheese
Avocado Spray

Instructions

1. Mix Birch Benders Keto Pancake and Waffle Mix with water and coconut oil according to package instructions.
2. Grease mini waffle iron with Avocado spray
3. Pour batter into waffle iron and cook according to iron Instructions.
4. While mini waffles are cooking (or before), scramble 2 eggs in small skillet.
5. Cook 3 strips of bacon (in an oven at 400 °F).
6. When mini waffles are done, let cool slightly on the plate or cooling rack.
7. When cooled, top two of the waffles with cheese slices, 1 1/2 bacon strips each, and divide the scrambled egg. Top with the remaining two mini waffles to make 2 sandwiches.
8. For a little extra spice, add Boars head honey mustard
9. Enjoy the breakfast sandwich!

Breakfast Pizza 11% (with 2 fiber caps)

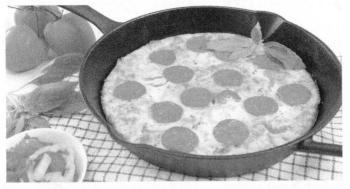

"Click Underlined Colored Word ingredients to buy them!

Ingredients

Cauliflower crust
free range eggs
mozzarella cheese
pizza seasoning to taste
Fresh Pressed Olive Oil

Instructions

1. Beat two eggs until they're well mixed.
2. Get your seasonings ready.
3. For this breakfast pizza I used thinly sliced green olives, thinly sliced black olives, pepperoni cut in half, and cubes of mozzarella.
4. Heat some olive oil in a porcelain pan over medium heat. Add the egg, season with pizza seasoning and oregano, and cook until eggs are about half set.
5. Then add half the pepperoni, olives, and mozzarella, followed by another layer of the four ingredients.
6. Be sure to end with cheese so there's some cheese on the top.
7. Cover the pan and cook 3-4 minutes, until eggs are not quite completely set.
8. Place all of the above on the cauliflower crust and then . . .
9. Place in the toaster-oven for about 4 minutes.
10. Delicious! pizza for breakfast!

Breakfast Mini Cheese Cake 11%
(with 2 fiber caps)

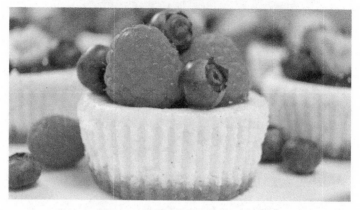

"Click Underlined Colored Word ingredients to buy them!"

Ingredients

Crust

2 cups whole almonds
2 tbsp. of liquid stevia
4 tbsp. salted Kerry butter

Filling

16 oz 4% fat cottage cheese
8 oz cream cheese
6 eggs
3/4 cup monk fruit powder
1/2 tsp almond extract
1/2 tsp vanilla extract

Topping

½ C of Blueberries
½ C of Raspberries

Instructions

1. Preheat the oven to 350. In a large food processor pulse the almonds, 2 tbsp. sweetener, and 4 tbsp. butter until a coarse dough forms. Grease two twelve hole standard silicone muffin pans or line metal tins with paper or foil cupcake liners. I used a silicone muffin pan for this and the cheesecakes popped out really easily. Divide the dough between the 24 holes and press into the bottom to form a crust. Bake for 8 minutes.

2. Meanwhile, combine the Friendship Dairies 4% cottage cheese and the cream cheese in the food processor (you don't need to wash the bowl). Pulse the cheeses until smooth. Add the sweetener and extracts. Mix until combined.

3. Add the eggs. Blend until smooth. You will need to scrape down the sides. Divide the batter between the muffin cups.

4. Bake for 30-40 minutes until the centers no longer jiggly when the pan is lightly shaken. Cool completely. Refrigerate for at least 2 hours before trying to remove them if you didn't use paper or foil liners.

5. Top with fresh blueberries and raspberries!

6. **Note:** This makes 24 individual cheesecakes. They freeze really well! I wrap them in plastic wrap and freeze them individually. To serve just thaw in the fridge overnight and then top with some berries. I eat two for breakfast or one as a snack.

Pepperoni Pizza Crustless Quiche 10%
(with 2 fiber caps)

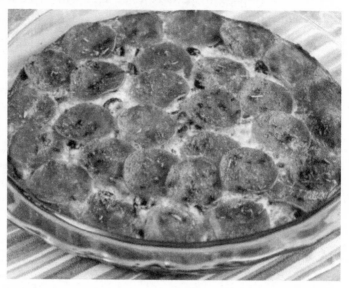

"Click <u>Underlined Colored Word</u> ingredients to buy them!"

Ingredients

8 oz. sliced mushrooms
2 tsp Fresh Pressed Olive Oil
1 2.25 oz. can sliced black olives, drained well
1 cup shredded Mozzarella cheese
1 cup shredded Goat cheese
1 tsp. + 1/2 tsp. Italian Herb blend
4 eggs, beaten well
1/2 cup heavy cream
1/4 tsp. garlic powder
2 oz. sliced pepperoni

Instructions

1. Preheat the oven to 400F/200C. Spray a 9 - 10 inch glass pie dish with non-stock spray.
2. Heat the olive oil in a non-stick frying pan. (I used my favorite 12" ceramic pan)
3. Add the sliced mushrooms and cook over medium-high heat until mushrooms release the liquid, the liquid evaporates, and mushrooms are cooked and lightly brown.

146

4. While mushrooms cook, dump olives into a colander placed in the sink and let them drain well.
5. Combine the Mozzarella and Goat Cheese in a bowl and sprinkle over the 1 tsp. Italian Herb Blend Stir the cheese with a fork so the dried herbs are evenly distributed in the cheese. Place the cheese in the pie dish.
6. Beat the eggs with a fork, then mix in the heavy cream, half and half, or milk and the garlic powder.
7. Mix the egg/cream mixture into the cheese in the pie dish, stirring well with a fork until all the cheese is completely coated with the egg mixture.
8. Make a layer of browned mushrooms on top of the cheese/egg mixture. Top that with the sliced olives if using.
9. Arrange the pepperoni slices in an overlapping layer over the top of the mushrooms and olives. Sprinkle with the other 1/2 teaspoon of Italian Herb Blend.
10. Bake the quiche 30-35 minutes, or until the eggs are completely set and the pepperoni is starting to brown.
11. Let it cool 3-5 minutes (it will sink down slightly as it cools. Serve hot.
12. This will keep for several days in the refrigerator and reheat well in the microwave or in a pan on the stove.

Lunch / Dinner

GREEN VEGGIES

Try to use some of them at every meal!!!
*Just remember to melt butter or Fresh Pressed Olive Oil
and dip them in it!
**If you don't use regenerative organic veggies
Always wash them with Veggie Wash or
Life Ionizer 11.5pH water!

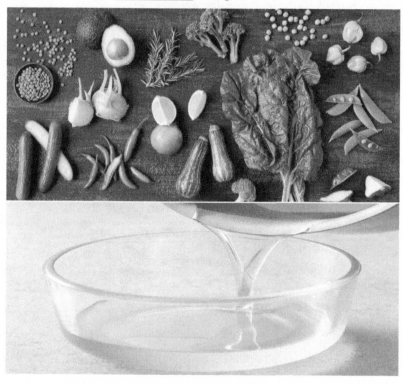

"Click Underlined Colored Word ingredients to buy them!"

Southern Fried Chicken 12% (with <u>2 fiber caps</u>)

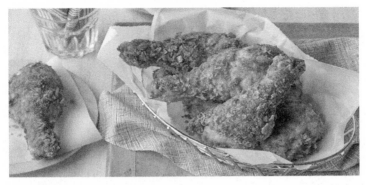

"Click <u>Underlined Colored Word</u> ingredients to buy them!"

Ingredients

12 chicken drumsticks or wings
4 cups unsweetened <u>almond milk</u>
4 tbsp. <u>lemon juice</u>
2 tbsp. <u>celtic sea salt</u>
2 tsp <u>ground black pepper</u>
2 tsp dried <u>oregano</u>
1 tsp <u>garlic powder</u>
1 tsp <u>onion powder</u>
1 ¼ cup pork rinds
¼ cup coconut flour
<u>coconut oil cooking spray</u>

Instructions

1. Combine almond milk, lemon juice, 2 tablespoons of salt, 1 teaspoon of pepper and 1 teaspoon of dried oregano in a bowl.
2. Submerge chicken pieces and leave to brine for a minimum of 90 minutes and a maximum of overnight.
3. Once brining is complete, add remaining ingredients, except cooking oil, into a food processor and pulse until combined into fine crumbs.
4. Preheat the oven to 400 °F (conventional). Shake crumbed coating out onto a tray. One at a time, remove chicken pieces from the brine solution and roll in coating until evenly coated.
5. Place coated pieces on a lined baking tray. Once all pieces are coated, bake for approx. 45 minutes depending on the size of

your pieces. Mid-way through the baking time, remove from the oven and spray with coconut oil cooking spray.

Butter Glazed Salmon & Asparagus 13% (with 2 fiber caps)

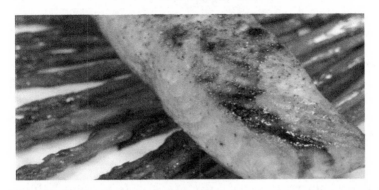

"Click <u>Underlined Colored Word</u> ingredients to buy them!"

Ingredients

½ cup of Kerry Butter
2 teaspoons Dijon mustard
1 teaspoon monk fruit liquid
2 4-oz salmon fillets
½ green onion, chopped

Instructions

1. Preheat the oven to 400 degrees. Combine butter, Dijon mustard, and monk fruit in a small saucepan and bring to a boil over medium heat. Simmer and cook for about 10 minutes or until the consistency is thick.
2. Use half of the butter glaze in brushing salmon fillet and in bottom of cast iron skillet
3. Fry in a cast iron skillet and glazed salmon fillets for 10-14 minutes.
4. Steam the asparagus for 10 to 15 minutes (until soft)
5. Remove baked salmon from the oven.
6. Pour the remaining glaze over salmon and asparagus
7. Top with green onion and serve hot.

Sausage and Pepperoni Pizza-Stuffed Peppers 14% (with 2 fiber caps)

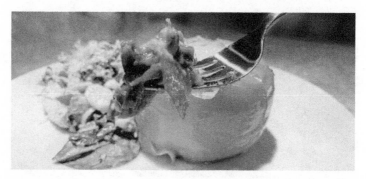

"Click Underlined Colored Word ingredients to buy them!"

Ingredients

19.5 oz Italian sausage or beyond meat sausage links
1 T olive oil
1 small onion, chopped
1 T minced garlic
14 oz. jar pizza sauce
2 tsp. dried oregano
3 large bell peppers, cut in half lengthwise and stem and seeds removed
3 oz. pepperoni
2 1/2 cups grated Mozzarella cheese
1 - 2 Tbsp. Fresh Pressed Olive Oil

Instructions

1. Preheat oven to 375F Spray a 9" x 13" casserole dish or large baking sheet with olive oil
2. Heat olive oil in a large non-stick frying pan over medium-high heat and squeeze sausage out of the casings and add to the pan, breaking apart with your fingers as you add it. Cook until sausage is nicely browned, breaking apart with a turner as it cooks.
3. While the sausage cooks, cut 12 pepperoni slices in halves and the rest into fourths. Grate cheese if needed, or measure out the desired amount of pre-grated cheese. Cut peppers in half and remove the seeds and cut out the stem end.

4. When the sausage is nicely browned, push it to the side and add the onions and garlic. Turn heat to medium and cook onions and garlic for 2-3 minutes.
5. Add the sauce and the dried oregano, turn heat to low, and simmer until the sauce is reduced and thickened.
6. Turn off heat, let the mixture cool for a few minutes, then add the chopped pepperoni and 2 cups grated Mozzarella, stirring gently so it's well-mixed with the sausage mixture.
7. Fill each pepper with the pizza-stuffing mixture, packing it in so all the stuffing is used.
8. Bake peppers for 20 minutes. Then remove from the oven and add a generous pinch of grated cheese and four pepperoni halves to the top of each pepper. Put back in the oven and bake 25 minutes more, or until the cheese is nicely browned, peppers are cooked, and the stuffing mixture is bubbling hot.

InsulThin Tuna Stuffed Avocado with Cilantro and Lime 13% (1 fiber cap)

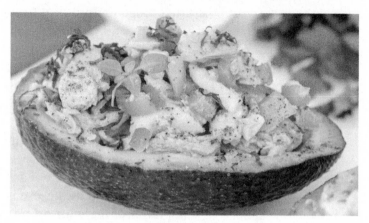

"Click Underlined Colored Word ingredients to buy them!"

Ingredients

1 plastic container wild caught tuna
1 large ripe avocado
1/4 cup very finely chopped red onion
1/2 cup fresh finely chopped cilantro
2 tsp. fresh Pressed Olive Oil
1 T Mayo
1 – 2 T fresh-squeezed lime juice (more or less to taste, see notes)
sea salt (or salt) and fresh ground black pepper to taste
additional lime for serving, if desired.

Instructions

1. Drain one can of tuna into a colander placed in the sink and gently break the tuna apart with a fork.
2. Finely chop red onion and cilantro. (You can use green onion instead of red onion if you prefer, especially if you are not using cilantro.)
3. Cut avocado in half.
4. Scrape out most of the avocado, leaving a tiny bit next to the skin to keep the shape of the avocado. Put avocado you removed into a large, flat bowl where you'll be able to easily mash avocado.

5. Use a large fork to thoroughly mash the avocado.
6. Then mix the olive oil, mayo, lime juice, salt, and pepper into the mashed avocado.
7. Mix the drained tuna into the avocado mixture.
8. Then gently stir in the chopped cilantro and red onion.
9. Season mixture to taste with salt and fresh-ground black pepper.
10. Stuff the mixture into the avocado halves and devour!
11. Serve with a generous wedge of lime to squeeze on at the table if desired

Meatball Casserole 14% (with 2 fiber caps)

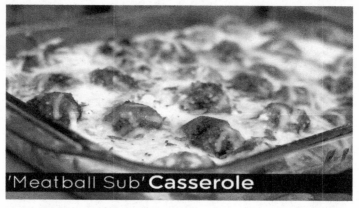

"Click <u>Underlined Colored Word</u> ingredients to buy them!"

Meatball Ingredients

1 lb. ground turkey
1 lb. Italian sausage
1 cup shredded mozzarella
1/3 cup grated or shredded parmesan
1 shredded zucchini about 1 cup
1 egg
2 tsp dried minced onion
2 tsp dried minced garlic
2 tsp dried basil
1 tsp celtic salt

Casserole Ingredients

1 cup **no sugar added pasta sauce**
8 oz shredded cheese (I used a two cheese pizza blend of mozzarella and provolone)

Instructions

1. Preheat the oven to 400. Spray a casserole dish with Coconut cooking spray
2. Combine all the ingredients for the meatballs and mix thoroughly. Make about 24 meatballs and put them in the casserole dish.

3. Bake for 30 minutes or until the meatballs are cooked through. Carefully drain the cooking liquid from the casserole dish.
4. Top with the sauce and cheese. Bake for an additional 10-15 minutes or until the cheese is melted.
5. Optional: I broiled for 3-4 minutes at the end to toast the cheese. Watch it carefully if you put it under the broiler. The cheese can burn easily.

Note-Substitutions: you can use any type of ground meat (beef, pork, turkey, chicken) and any type of Italian sausage (pork, chicken, or turkey) in these meatballs

Nacho Steak Skillet 14% (with 2 fiber caps)

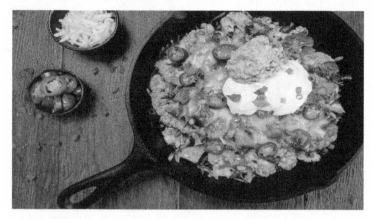

"Click <u>Underlined Colored Word</u> ingredients to buy them!"

Ingredients

8 ounces beef round tip steak, thinly sliced*
1 tablespoon <u>Kerry butter</u>
1/3 cup refined <u>coconut oil</u>. melted
1 teaspoon <u>chili powder</u>
½ teaspoon <u>turmeric</u>
1lb 8oz cauliflower
1 ounce shredded <u>cheddar cheese</u>
1 ounce shredded <u>Monterey jack</u>
30 g canned <u>jalapeño slices</u>
1/3 cup sour cream
136 g avocado
1-2 Tbsp. <u>Fresh Pressed Olive Oil</u>

Instructions

1. Preheat your oven to 400°F. Remove the leaves and bottom of the stem from your cauliflower. Slice the cauliflower across the head. It will break up into chip-like shapes.
2. In the bottom of a large mixing bowl whisk together the coconut oil, chili powder, and turmeric. Add the cauliflower and gently toss until it's all evenly coated.
3. Spread the cauliflower out on a baking sheet. Season well with salt and pepper. Roast for 20-25 minutes.
4. While the cauliflower is roasting you can get the rest of it ready. Preheat a cast iron skillet on medium-high heat.

Liberally season both sides of your steak with salt and pepper. Add the olive oil to the skillet and let it melt. Once it stops foaming, lay the steak down into the pan. Cook without disturbing until it begins to cook through. Flip to cook the other side then remove from the pan.

5. Allow to rest for 5-10 minutes.
6. Once the cauliflower is done, remove it from the oven and transfer the florets to your cast iron pan.
7. Slice up the steak into fork sized strips.
8. Top the cauliflower with the steak.
9. Top the skillet with both shredded cheeses and the jalapeño slices. Bake for another 5-10 minutes, until the cheese has melted.
10. Serve with sour cream, guacamole, and hot sauce. You can garnish with cilantro and slices of green onion if you desire.

Shrimp Avocado Salad 13%
(with 2 fiber caps)

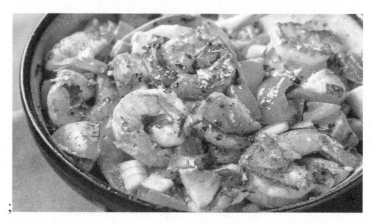

;

"Click Underlined Colored Word ingredients to buy them!"

A delicious, low carb cold shrimp salad with avocado, tomatoes, feta cheese, and lemon juice.

Ingredients

8 ounces shrimp peeled, deveined, patted dry
1 large avocado diced
1 small beefsteak tomato diced and drained
1/3 cup crumbled feta cheese
1/3 cup freshly chopped cilantro or parsley
2 tablespoons salted butter melted
1 tablespoon lemon juice
1 tablespoon fresh pressed olive oil
1/4 teaspoon Celtic sea salt
1/4 teaspoon black pepper

Instructions

1. Toss shrimp with melted butter in a bowl until well-coated.
2. Heat a pan over medium-high heat for a few minutes until hot. Add shrimp to the pan in a single layer, searing for a minute or until it starts to become pink around the edges, then flip and cook until shrimp are cooked through, less than a minute.

3. Transfer the shrimp to a plate as they finish cooking. Let them cool while you prepare the other ingredients.
4. Add all other ingredients to a large mixing bowl -- diced avocado, diced tomato, feta cheese, cilantro, lemon juice, olive oil, salt, and pepper -- and toss to mix.
5. Add shrimp and stir to mix together. Add additional salt and pepper to taste.

Sweet Onion Frittata 12% (with <u>2 fiber caps)</u>

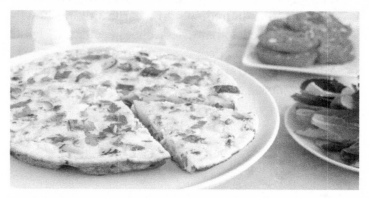

"Click <u>Underlined Colored Word</u> ingredients to buy them!"

Ingredients

4 ounces chopped extra lean, ham slices
1 cup Vidalia or Texas Sweet onion, thinly sliced
1 ½ cups liquid whole egg
½ cup shredded, <u>sharp cheddar cheese</u>
Fresh on the vine tomatoes
1-2 tbsp. <u>fresh pressed olive oil</u>

Instructions

1. Place a medium porcelain skillet over medium-high heat until hot and then coat with olive oil
2. Cook ham for about 2-3 minutes, or until lightly brown. Remove from the skillet and set aside.
3. Coat skillet with olive oil. Cook onions for about 4 minutes, or until golden. Add ham and cook for another minute, allowing the flavors to blend.
4. Pour egg substitute evenly, cover and cook for about 8 minutes or until puffy and set.
5. Remove the skillet from the heat. Sprinkle cheese on top, cover and let stand for about 3 minutes until the cheese melts.
6. Slice tomatoes and sprinkle celtic sea salt on - serve on the side.

Turkey Bacon Ranch Pinwheels 14%
(with 2 fiber caps)

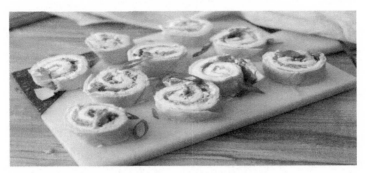

"Click Underlined Colored Word ingredients to buy them!"

Ingredients

6 oz cream cheese
12 slices smoked deli turkey about 3 oz
1/4 tsp each garlic powder dill, and minced onion
1 tbsp. bacon crumbles
2 tbsp. finely shredded cheddar cheese

Instructions

1. Put the cream cheese between 2 pieces of plastic wrap. Roll it out until it's about 1/4 inch thick. Peel off the top piece of plastic wrap. Lay the slices of turkey on top of the cream cheese.
2. Cover with a new piece of plastic wrap and flip the whole thing over. Peel off the piece of plastic that is now on the top. Sprinkle the spices on top of the cream cheese. Sprinkle with the bacon and cheese.
3. Roll up the pinwheels so that the turkey is on the outside. Refrigerate for at least 2 hours. Thinly slice and serve on top of low carb crackers or sliced cucumber.

Chicken Salad Lettuce Wraps 14%
(with 2 fiber caps)

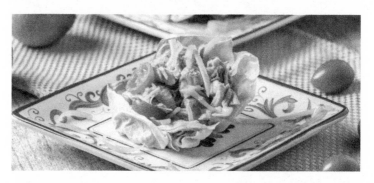

"Click Underlined Colored Word ingredients to buy them!"

Ingredients

1.5 lb. chicken breast
3 ribs celery, diced
1/2 cup **mayo**
2 tsp Boars Head Honey Mustard
1/2 tsp pink Himalayan salt
2 tbsp. fresh dill, chopped
1/4 cup chopped pecans
Romaine lettuce
Cherry tomatoes

Instructions

1. Preheat oven to 450°F and line baking sheet with parchment paper.
2. Bake chicken breast until cooked throughout, about 15 minutes.
3. Remove chicken from the oven and let it cool. After completely cooled, cut chicken into bite-sized pieces.
4. In a large bowl, add chicken, celery, mayo, brown mustard, and salt. Toss until chicken is fully coated and ingredients are well-combined.
5. Cover bowl with lid or plastic wrap and refrigerate until chilled, about 1-2 hours.
6. When ready to serve, place in one romaine leaf and top with sliced cherry tomatoes.

Chicken Alfredo Spaghetti Squash 14% (with 2 fiber caps)

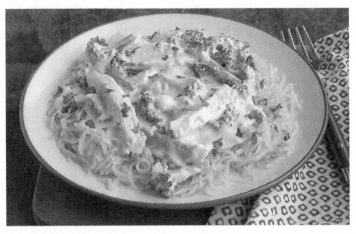

"Click <u>Underlined Colored Word</u> ingredients to buy them!"

Ingredients

1 spaghetti squash (2 lb.)
2-1/2 cups small broccoli florets
2 Tbsp. Italian Dressing
1 lb. boneless skinless chicken breasts, cut into strips
2 tsp. Almond flour
1 cup chicken broth
4 oz. (1/2 of 8-oz. pkg.) PHILADELPHIA Cheese, cubed
1/2 cup Shredded Parmesan Cheese
1/8 tsp. each black pepper and ground nutmeg

Instructions

1. Pierce squash in several places with a sharp knife or fork; place in a shallow microwaveable dish. Microwave on HIGH 10 to 15 min. or until squash is softened, turning every 5 min. Cool slightly.

2. Meanwhile, place broccoli in a microwaveable bowl. Add enough water to cover broccoli. Microwave 3 to 4 min. or until broccoli is crisp-tender; drain.3

3. Heat dressing in a large nonstick skillet on medium heat. Add chicken; cook 4 to 5 min. or until done, stirring occasionally.

Remove chicken from skillet, reserving drippings in skillet; cover chicken to keep warm.4

4. Whisk flour and broth until blended. Add to drippings in the skillet along with remaining ingredients; stir. Cook for 2 min. or until sauce comes to a boil, stirring constantly to scrape browned bits from the bottom of the skillet. Cook and stir 1 to 2 min. or until thickened.5

5. Return chicken to skillet along with the broccoli; cook 1 to 2 min. or until heated through, stirring frequently.6

6. Cut squash in half; remove and discard seeds. Use a fork to scrape insides of squash into strands; place in a bowl. Serve topped with chicken mixture.

Zucchini With Mozzarella and Pepperoni 12% (with 2 fiber caps)

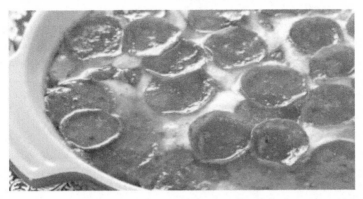

"Click <u>Underlined Colored Word</u> ingredients to buy them!"

Ingredients

3-4 zucchini, 8-10 inches long (same size zucchini works best)
1 tsp. Spike Seasoning
1 tsp. Italian Herb Blend
about 3/4 lb. grated mozzarella
about 20 slices pepperoni, cut in half

Instructions

1. Preheat broiler and put rack into middle position or about 4 inches away from broiler.
2. Wash zucchini and cut off the ends.
3. Cut into slices about 3/8 inches wide, using a **mandolin** if you have one. It's important that all zucchini slices are the same width so they can cook evenly.
4. Spray a large baking sheet with non-stick spray.
5. Cover the baking sheet completely with zucchini rounds, putting them as close together as possible.
6. Sprinkle each zucchini piece with **Spike Seasoning** and **Italian Herb Blend** Completely cover top of zucchini with grated cheese.
7. Broil until the cheese is starting to melt, about 3 minutes.

8. Cut pepperoni slices in half while the cheese is starting to melt, then sprinkle the cut pepperoni slices over the partially melted cheese.

9. Broil about 3-4 minutes more, or until the pepperoni is slightly crisped and the cheese is starting to brown. Serve immediately.

Beyond Meat Butter Crusted Burgers 11% (with <u>2 fiber caps</u>)

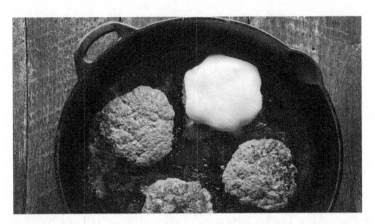

"Click <u>Underlined Colored Word</u> ingredients to buy them!"

Ingredients

½ stick of <u>Kerry butter</u>
1 small Vidalia or red onion
1 pinch of <u>Celtic sea salt</u>
2 pieces of your favorite cheese

Instructions

1. Heat on high a seasoned black cast iron pan.
2. Place Kerry butter in the pan and then put red or Vidalia onion in.
3. take beyond meat burgers and generously shake Dr. Paul's Blackened seasoning on them.
4. Place burgers in a pan and sauté until caramelized. Then place your beyond meat burgers in the pan. Cook until brown on each side.
5. Add your favorite cheese until it melts.
6. Serve quickly and you will eat quickly too because they are sooo good!!

Spicy Dry Rub Chicken Wings 14%
(with 2 fiber caps)

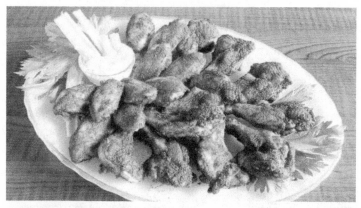

"Click Underlined Colored Word ingredients to buy them!"

Ingredients

2 pounds chicken wings about 20 wings & drumettes
1 tablespoon fresh pressed olive oil
1 tablespoon chili powder
1 tablespoon smoked paprika
1 1/2 teaspoons ground cumin
1 teaspoon ground cayenne pepper more for hotter wings
1 1/2 teaspoons garlic powder
1 1/2 teaspoons onion powder
1 1/2 teaspoons Real salt
1 1/2 teaspoons black pepper

Instructions

1. Dry wing pieces with paper towels to remove excess liquid.
2. Place wings in a large bowl and rub olive oil evenly into each piece.
3. Combine all seasonings in a bowl.
4. Sprinkle half of the season mix onto the chicken wings and rub in. Flip wings and sprinkle remaining half onto wings and rub in.
5. Place rack over shallow baking pan with sides (line pan with foil for easy cleanup). Place seasoned wings on the rack.
6. Bake at 350 degrees °F for 20 minutes, flip each wing, then bake for an additional 10 minutes.

7. Turn the oven broiler on low and broil for another 10 minutes.
8. Remove from the oven. Serve with celery and blue cheese dressing if desired.

Cheesy Taco Casserole 12% (with 2 fiber caps)

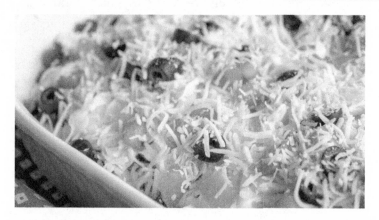

"Click Underlined Colored Word ingredients to buy them!"

Ingredients

1 Taco Tuesday
3 lbs. 80/20 Ground Beef or a package of beyond meat crumbles
2 Cups Pepper Jack Cheese (Shredded)
4 Cups Colby & Monterey Jack Cheese (Shredded)
2 Cups Frozen Pepper Strips (Green, Red, and Yellow) thawed
4 oz black olives
1 on the vine roma tomato1
1-2 tbsp. fresh pressed olive oil

Instructions

1. Preheat oven to 350.
2. Brown ground beef in a large skillet and drain (set aside).
3. Sauté peppers in 1-2 tablespoons of olive oil.
4. Cut up olives and tomato.
5. Mix ground beef and peppers together and pour into the bottom of a 9 x 13 pan.
6. Top meat mixture with cheese and bake for 10 min. and broil for 5 minutes until golden brown

Chicken Bacon Ranch Casserole 13% (with 2 fiber caps)

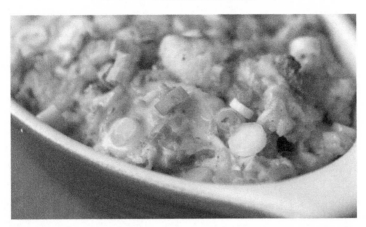

"Click Underlined Colored Word ingredients to buy them!"

Ingredients

Chicken breast – either cubed baked chicken or shredded chicken
Scallions
Bacon
Ranch dressing
Fresh pressed olive oil

Instructions

1. Bacon – cooked until crispy, either on the stove or bacon in the oven Garlic – minced
2. Ranch dressing
3. Vegetables – fresh or frozen
4. Shredded cheese
5. Cook your broccoli or other veggies in olive oil.
6. Mix all the ingredients together in a large bowl, reserving half of the shredded cheeses.
7. Transfer your easy casserole mixture to a baking dish and top with the remaining cheese.
8. Baking time takes only about 15 minutes, just until the chicken bacon casserole is hot and bubbly. Viola! This will be one of your favorite low carb meals for a busy weeknights.

Bacon Wrapped Cheese Stuffed Burgers 14%
(with 2 fiber caps)

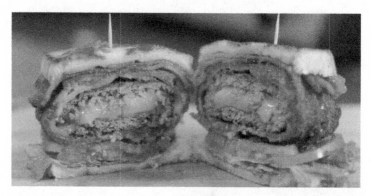

"Click Underlined Colored Word ingredients to buy them!"

Ingredients

Filling

2 tbsp. ghee
1 medium white onion, sliced (110 g/ 4 oz)
2 ¹/₂ cups sliced bell peppers (225 g/ 8 oz)
2 cups sliced white mushrooms (140 g/ 5 oz)

Burgers

2 lbs. ground beef or Beyond Meat ground
salt & pepper to taste
10 thin-cut slices bacon (150 g/ 5.3 oz)
1 ¹/₄ cups shredded cheddar cheese (140 g/ 5 oz)
5 tsp *Sriracha*
5 tsp *Dijon mustard*

Instructions

1. Grease a large pan with ghee. Once hot, add sliced onion and cook over a medium-high heat for 5 minutes or until lightly browned.
2. Add sliced bell peppers and cook for another 5 minutes.
3. Add sliced mushrooms and cook for 3-5 minutes. Take off the heat

4. Use your hands to divide the ground beef into 5 parts (200 grams or 7.1 ounces each). Flatten each part using your hands. Then take a glass and place in the middle of the burger to create a well. Fold the meat up round the glass to create a bowl shape.
5. Wrap 2 slices of bacon round the "meat bowl". Then, remove the glass carefully by gently twisting and pulling it up.
6. Fill each "meat bowl" with the onion-pepper-mushroom mixture and a teaspoon of Sriracha and Dijon mustard.
7. Finally, top with $1/4$ cup of grated cheese. Repeat for the remaining burgers.
8. Place in the oven and bake at 150 °C/ 300 °F for 45-60 minutes (until the meat thermometer registers 75 °C/ 165 °F). When done, remove from the oven and let the burgers rest for 5 minutes.
9. Place in Zero Carb bread with Dijon Mustard with lettuce.
10. Serve with crispy greens or other low-carb veggies.

Grilled Skirt Steak 14% (with 2 fiber caps)

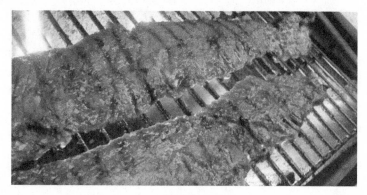

"Click Underlined Colored Word ingredients to buy them!"

1 1/2 lb. skirt steak

2 tsp. cumin

1 tsp. coriander

2 garlic cloves, minced

4 tbsp. lime juice

3 tbsp. Fresh pressed olive oil

3 avocados, diced

2 tbsp. finely chopped red onion

2 tbsp. finely chopped fresh cilantro, plus cilantro leaves for serving

1/2 tsp. crushed red pepper flakes

3/4 c. red grape tomatoes, halved

3/4 c. yellow grape tomatoes, halved

Celtic sea salt

Freshly ground black pepper

Instructions

1. Place steak in a shallow glass baking dish.
2. In a small bowl, whisk together cumin, coriander, garlic, 2 tablespoons lime juice, and 2 tablespoons olive oil. Pour mixture over steak, turning to coat, and marinate 10 minutes.

176

3. Make guacamole: In a medium bowl, mash together avocado, onion, cilantro, red pepper flakes, and remaining 2 tablespoons lime juice until chunky, then season with salt.
4. In a medium bowl, mix tomatoes with remaining 1 tablespoon olive oil and season with salt and pepper.
5. Heat a grill pan over medium-high heat.
6. Grill tomatoes until blistered, 4 minutes, then remove tomatoes and increase heat to high.
7. Add steak to grill and season with salt and pepper. Grill 3 minutes per side for medium-rare, then let sit 5 minutes.
8. Thinly slice steak against the grain. Top with blistered tomatoes and cilantro, and serve with guacamole.

Chicken Tikka Masala 14%(with 2 fiber caps)

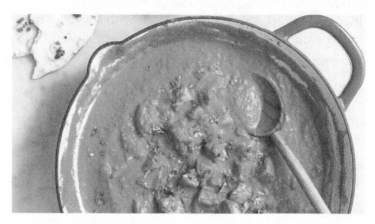

"Click Underlined Colored Word ingredients to buy them!"

Ingredients

For the chicken marinade

28 oz (800g) boneless and skinless chicken thighs cut into bite-sized pieces

1 cup plain yogurt

1 1/2 tablespoons fresh minced garlic

1 tablespoon fresh ginger

2 teaspoons garam masala

1 teaspoon turmeric

1 teaspoon ground cumin

1 teaspoon Kashmiri chili

1 teaspoon of Celtic salt

Monk fruit powder

For the sauce

2 tablespoons of fresh pressed olive oil

2 tablespoons Kerry butter

2 small onions (or 1 large onion) finely diced

1 1/2 tablespoons garlic finely grated

1 tablespoon ginger finely grated

1 1/2 teaspoons garam masala

1 1/2 teaspoons ground cumin

1 teaspoon turmeric powder

1 teaspoon ground coriander

14 oz (400g) tomato puree

1 teaspoon Kashmiri chili

1 teaspoon ground red chili powder (adjust to your taste preference)

1 teaspoon Celtic salt

1 1/4 cups of heavy cream

1 teaspoon Monk fruit powder

1/4 cup Alkaline water (Evian)

4 tablespoons Fresh cilantro or coriander to garnish.

Instructions

1. In a bowl, combine chicken with all of the ingredients for the chicken marinade; let marinate for 10 minutes to an hour (or overnight if time allows).

2. Heat oil in a large skillet or pot over medium-high heat. When sizzling, add chicken pieces in batches of two or three, making sure not to crowd the pan. Fry until browned for only 3 minutes on each side. Set aside and keep warm. (You will finish cooking the chicken in the sauce.)

3. Melt the butter in the same pan. Fry the onions until soft (about 3 minutes) while scraping up any browned bits stuck on the bottom of the pan.

4. Add garlic and ginger and sauté for 1 minute until fragrant, then add garam masala, cumin, turmeric and coriander. Fry for about 20 seconds until fragrant, while stirring occasionally.

5. Pour in the tomato puree, chili powders and salt. Let simmer for about 10-15 minutes, stirring occasionally until sauce thickens and becomes a deep brown red color.

6. Stir the cream and sugar through the sauce. Add the chicken and its juices back into the pan and cook for an additional 8-10 minutes until chicken is cooked through and the sauce is thick and bubbling. Pour in the water to thin out the sauce, if needed.

7. Garnish with cilantro (coriander) and serve with fresh, hot cauliflower rice.
8. Fried lavash bread and Kerry butter

InsulThin Soups and Salads

Fresh Vegetable Soup 10% (1 fiber cap)

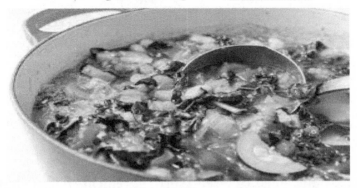

"Click <u>Underlined Colored Word</u> ingredients to buy them!"

Ingredients

1 cup cauliflower

1 small onion

1 small bone broth

1 stalk celery

1 cup broccoli

3 stalks asparagus (or tinned)

1 liter Life Ionizer water / Evian water

4 teaspoons yeast-free vegetable broth

1 tsp fresh basil

2 tsp celtic sea salt to taste.

Instructions

1. Put the water into a pot, add vegetable broth and chopped onion, and bring to boil.
2. Finely chop basil and asparagus, and shred cauliflower and celery in the food processor. Once water has boiled add the vegetables and leave in boiling water until tender. Allow to cool, then add ingredients to a blender and mix until it is a thick, smooth consistency

Broccoli Cheese Soup 12%(with 2 fiber caps)

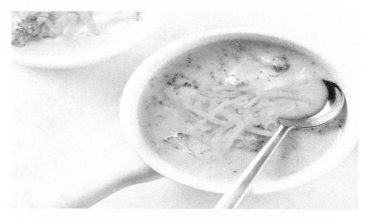

"Click <u>Underlined Colored Word</u> ingredients to buy them!"

Ingredients

Broccoli Garlic fresh
Heavy Coconut cream
Fresh pressed olive oil
Chicken broth
Shredded cheddar cheese

Instructions

1. Sauté garlic in olive oil in a large pot or Dutch oven. It takes about 45-60 seconds, until fragrant.
2. Add chicken broth, heavy cream, and chopped broccoli. Simmer until the broccoli is tender, about 10-20 minutes. TIP: The simmer time will vary depending on the size of your florets. Smaller florets = faster simmer time.
3. Add the shredded cheddar cheese gradually, stirring constantly, and continue to stir until melted. This will help thicken the soup. TIP: Avoid having the heat too high when adding the cheese or after, to avoid seizing.
4. OR, to avoid clumping together…Puree the broccoli into the soup along with the cheddar cheese using an immersion blender. I like to remove about 1/3 the florets using a slotted spoon first, so that you can toss the florets back in afterward and have some broccoli pieces in your soup. TIP: The more broccoli you leave in before pureeing, the thicker your broccoli

soup will be. The cheese helps thicken your broccoli cheddar soup, but the pureed broccoli florets will, too!

5. this low carb broccoli cheese soup recipe has just 4g net carbs and 5g total carbs.

Chili 12%(with 2 fiber caps)

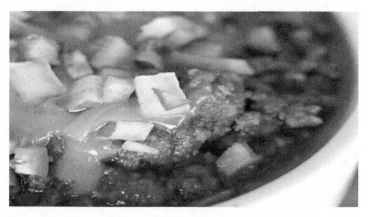

"Click Underlined Colored Word ingredients to buy them!"

Ingredients

3 slices bacon, cut into 1/2" strips
1/4 medium yellow onion, chopped
2 celery stalks, chopped
1 green bell pepper, chopped
1/2 c. sliced baby Bellas
2 cloves garlic, minced
2 lb. ground beef or Beyond Meat
2 tbsp. chili powder
2 tsp. ground turmeric
2 tsp. dried oregano
2 tbsp. smoked paprika
Celtic salt
Freshly ground black pepper
Fresh pressed olive oil
2 c. low-sodium beef broth
Sour cream, for garnish
Shredded cheddar, for garnish
Sliced green onions, for garnish
Sliced avocado, for garnish

Instructions

1. In a large pot over medium heat, cook bacon. When bacon is crisp, remove from the pot with a slotted spoon.
2. Add onion, celery, pepper, and mushrooms to pot and cook until soft, 6 minutes.
3. Add garlic and cook until fragrant, 1 minute more.
4. Push vegetables to one side of the pan and add beef. Cook, stirring occasionally, until no pink remains. Drain fat and return to heat.
5. Add chili powder, cumin, oregano, and paprika and season with salt and pepper. Stir to combine and cook 2 minutes more.
6. Add broth and bring to a simmer. Let cook for 10 to 15 more minutes, until most of the broth has evaporated.
7. Ladle into bowls and top with sour cream, reserved bacon, cheese, green onions, and avocado.

Thai Chicken Coconut Soup 12% (with 2 fiber caps)

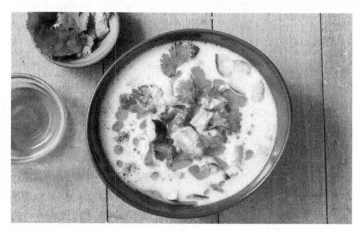

"Click **Underlined Colored Word** ingredients to buy them!"

Ingredients

1 tbsp. Fresh pressed olive oil
1 tbsp. freshly minced ginger
4 oz. shiitake mushrooms, chopped
6 c. chicken broth low-sodium chicken broth
1 (14-oz.) can) coconut milk
1 tbsp. fish sauce
1 lb. boneless skinless chicken thighs, cut into 1" pieces
Juice of 1 lime
Fresh Cilantro leaves, for garnish

Instructions

1. In a large pot over medium heat, heat oil. Add ginger and cook until fragrant, 1 minute, then add mushrooms and cook until soft, about 6 minutes.
2. Add broth, coconut milk, and fish sauce and bring to a boil. Add chicken, reduce heat, and simmer until chicken is no longer pink, about 15 minutes.
3. Turn off heat and stir in lime juice.
4. Garnish with cilantro and chili oil (if using) before serving

Baby Kale Avocado Salad 6% (with 2 fiber caps)

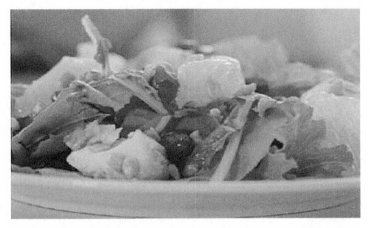

"Click Underlined Colored Word ingredients to buy them!"

Ingredients

10 oz Baby kale
1/4 cup fresh pressed olive oil
2 tbsp. lemon juice
2 cloves Garlic (minced)
1/4 tsp Celtic sea salt
1/4 tsp black pepper
1/2 cup Parmesan cheese (shaved or shredded)
1 medium Avocado (cubed)

Instructions

1. Place the chopped kale into a large bowl. Set aside.
2. In a small bowl, whisk together the olive oil, lemon juice, minced garlic, sea salt, and black pepper, until a dressing forms. (Alternatively, place dressing ingredients into an airtight container and shake vigorously.)
3. Pour the dressing over the kale leaves and toss to coat. Use your hands to massage the dressing into the leaves for a minute or two (pick up a bunch, squeeze, and repeat). Do this until the kale softens and begins to wilt. (It will happen fast with baby kale, and takes a little longer with regular kale.)
4. Add the parmesan cheese, chopped avocado,. Toss again.

Seriously, this is the easiest kale avocado salad recipe, plus the baby kale makes it much more approachable than most.

Instant Pot Taco Soup 11%(with 2 fiber caps)

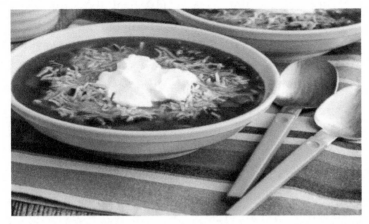

"Click <u>Underlined Colored Word</u> ingredients to buy them!"

Ingredients

2 lbs. <u>ground beef</u> or Beyond Meat (vegetarian)

1 T <u>fresh pressed olive oil</u>

<u>Celtic salt</u> and fresh-ground black pepper to taste

1 small onion, chopped small

1 red bell pepper, chopped small

1 Poblano pepper, chopped small (see notes)

1 T minced garlic (garlic from a jar is fine for this)

2 T <u>ground cumin</u>

1 T <u>Ground Chile Pepper</u>

1 T <u>chili powder</u>

<u>Celtic salt</u> and fresh-ground black pepper to taste

1 Fresh Avocado

Sour Cream or Tofutti Sour cream

<u>Mexican Cheese</u>

3 14 oz. cans beef broth (see notes)

2 14.5 oz cans petite diced tomatoes

1 T Sriracha <u>sauce</u>

2 T fresh-squeezed or fresh-frozen lime juice, to add at the end (more or less to taste)

Instructions

1. Turn Instant Pot to SAUTE, heat the olive oil for 1-2 minutes, then add the ground beef and cook until the beef is fully browned, breaking apart with the turner as it cooks and seasoning to taste with salt and fresh-ground black pepper.
2. While the beef cooks, chop the onion, red bell pepper, into small pieces.
3. When the meat is fully browned, add the minced garlic, .chili powder
4. Stir spices into the meat and cook 1-2 minutes; then add the chopped onion, red bell pepper, and Poblano pepper and cook 2-3 minutes more.
5. Add the beef broth and petite diced tomatoes with juice and stir.
6. Lock the lid on the Instant Pot, set to MANUAL with HIGH pressure and 10 minutes cooking time.
7. When ten minutes is up, let the pressure release naturally for about 20 minutes, then use the quick release method to release the rest of the pressure.
8. Check the soup to see if you think there is too much liquid and if so, use the SAUTE setting to cook for a few minutes and evaporate some of the liquid.
9. Stir in Sirach sauce and fresh-squeezed lime juice and Serve hot, with diced avocado, grated Mexican Blend Cheese, Sour cream, cut limes, and Sirach Sauce to add at the table if desired.

Egg Salad 11%(with 2 fiber caps)

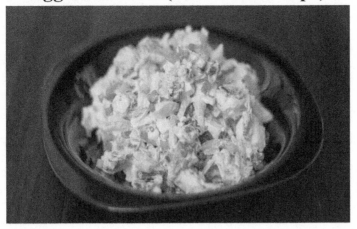

"Click <u>Underlined Colored Word</u> ingredients to buy them!"

Ingredients

3 tbsp. <u>mayonnaise</u>

2 tsp. lemon

1 tbsp. finely chopped chives

Freshly ground black pepper

<u>Celtic salt</u>

6 hard boiled eggs, peeled and chopped

1 avocado, cubed

Lettuce, for serving

Cooked <u>bacon</u>, for serving

Instructions

1. In a medium bowl, whisk together mayonnaise, lemon juice, and chives. Season with salt and pepper.
2. Add eggs and avocado and toss gently to combine.
3. Serve with lettuce and bacon

Grilled Chicken Salad 13% (2 fiber caps)

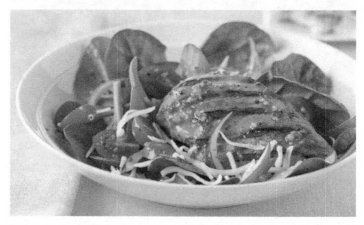

"Click Underlined Colored Word ingredients to buy them!"

Ingredients

2 boneless skinless chicken breasts (about 1 1/4 pounds)

1 tsp. ground coriander

1 tsp. oregano

Celtic salt

Freshly ground black pepper

5 tbsp. fresh pressed olive oil

4 tbsp. red wine vinegar

1 tbsp. freshly chopped parsley

4 romaine hearts, chopped

3 Persian cucumbers, thinly sliced

1 c. grape or cherry tomatoes, halved

2 avocados, sliced

4 oz. feta, crumbled

1/2 c. pitted Kalamata olives, halved

½ Red or Vidalia Onion

Cobb Egg Salad 12% (with 2 fiber caps)

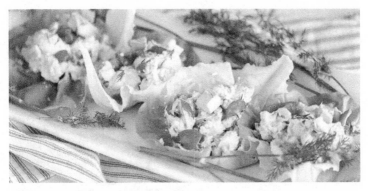

"Click Underlined Colored Word ingredients to buy them!"

Ingredients

3 tbsp. mayonnaise
3 tbsp. Coconut Cream
2 tbsp. red wine vinegar
Celtic salt
Freshly ground black pepper
8 hard-boiled eggs, cut into eight pieces, plus more for garnish
8 strips bacon, cooked and crumbled, plus more for garnish
1 avocado, thinly sliced
1/2 c. crumbled blue cheese, plus more for garnish
1/2 c. cherry tomatoes, halved, plus more for garnish
2 tbsp. freshly chopped chives
1 head romaine lettuce

Instructions

1. In a small bowl, stir together mayonnaise, yogurt, and red wine vinegar. Season with salt and pepper.
2. In a large serving bowl, gently mix together eggs, bacon, avocado, blue cheese, and cherry tomatoes. Gradually fold in mayonnaise dressing, using only enough until ingredients are lightly coated, then season with salt and pepper. Garnish with chives and additional toppings.
3. Serve on a leaf of romaine lettuce.

Shrimp de Gallo 13% (with 2 fiber caps)

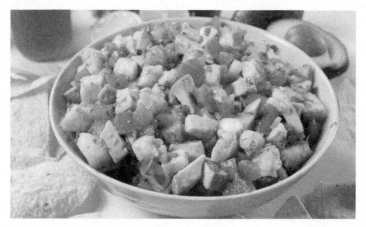

"Click <u>Underlined Colored Word</u> ingredients to buy them!"

Ingredients

<u>Keto chips</u> for serving 1 tbsp. <u>fresh pressed olive oil</u>
1 clove garlic, minced
1/4 tsp. <u>chili powder</u>
1 lb. large shrimp, tails removed
<u>Celtic salt</u>
1 1/2 lb. tomatoes, seeded and finely diced (about 3 cups)
1/2 c. finely chopped white onion
1/2 c. finely chopped cilantro
2 jalapeño peppers, seeds removed and finely diced
1 <u>avocado,</u>, finely diced
2 tbsp. fresh lime juice

Instructions

1. In a large skillet, heat oil over medium-high. Season shrimp with salt and add to skillet along with garlic and chili powder. Season with salt. Cook, tossing occasionally, until shrimp are pink and just cooked through, about 3 minutes. Using a slotted spoon, transfer shrimp to a cutting board to cool.

2. Roughly chop shrimp into small pieces and scrape into a medium bowl. Add tomatoes, onion, cilantro, jalapeños, lime juice, and avocado, and season with salt.
3. Mix until combined and serve with tortilla chips.

Chicken Salad Stuffed Avocados 14%
(with 2 fiber caps)

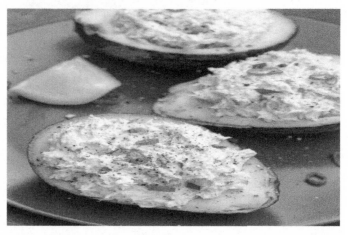

"Click Underlined Colored Word ingredients to buy them!"

Ingredients

2 avocados, pitted
2 c. shredded rotisserie chicken
1/4 c. red onion, minced
1/3 c. mayonnaise
2 tbsp. Greek yogurt
Juice of 1 lemon
1 1/2 tsp. Dijon mustard
celtic salt
Freshly ground black pepper
Chopped parsley, for garnish

Instructions

1. Scoop out avocados, leaving a small border. Dice avocado and set aside.
2. Make chicken salad: In a large bowl, mix together chicken, onion, mayo, Greek yogurt, lemon juice, and mustard. Fold in diced avocado. Season with salt and pepper.
3. Divide salad among 4 avocado halves.
4. Garnish with parsley.

Antipasto Salad 8% (1 fiber cap)

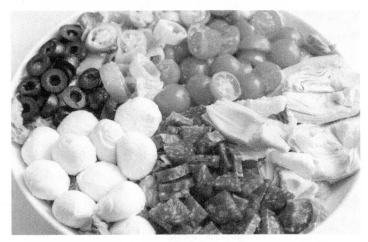

"Click <u>Underlined Colored Word</u> ingredients to buy them!"

Ingredients

For the salad

2 large romaine hearts, chopped
1/2 lb. salami
8 oz. mozzarella balls, halved
1 c. quartered artichoke hearts
1 c. cherry tomatoes, halved
1 c. chopped pepperoncini
1/2 c. sliced olives

For the red wine vinaigrette

1/2 c fresh press olive oil
1/4 c. red wine vinegar
1 tsp. Dijon mustard
1/2 tsp. oregano
1/4 tsp. red pepper flakes
celtic salt
Freshly ground black pepper

Instructions

1. In a large bowl toss lettuce, salami, mozzarella, artichokes, tomatoes, pepperoncini together.

2. Make the vinaigrette: In a jar fitted with a lid, shake together olive oil, vinegar, mustard, oregano, and red pepper flakes. Season with salt and pepper. Dress salad with vinaigrette and serve.

Greek Salad 13%(with 2 fiber caps)

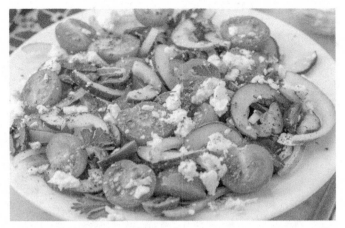

"Click Underlined Colored Word ingredients to buy them!"

Ingredients

For the salad

1 pt. grape or cherry tomatoes halved
1 cucumber, thinly sliced into half-moons
1 c. halved Kalamata olives
1/2 red onion, thinly sliced
3/4 c. crumbled feta

For the dressing

2 tbsp. apple
Juice of 1/2 a lemon
1 tsp. dried oregano
Celtic sea salt
Freshly ground black pepper
1/4 c. extra-virgin olive oil

Instructions

1. Make the salad: In a large bowl, stir together tomatoes, cucumber, olives, and red onion.
2. Gently fold in feta.
3. In a small bowl, make the dressing: Combine vinegar, lemon juice, and oregano and season with salt and pepper.
4. Slowly add olive oil, whisking to combine.
5. Drizzle dressing over salad.

Strawberry Spinach Salad 14%
(with 2 fiber caps)

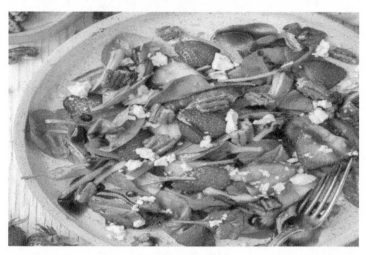

"Click Underlined Colored Word ingredients to buy them!"

Ingredients

2 tbsp. fresh lemon juice

1/2 tsp. Dijon mustard

1/4 c. fresh pressed olive oil

Celtic salt

Freshly ground black pepper

5 c. packed baby spinach (5 oz.)

2 rotisserie chicken breasts, cut into 1/2" pieces

2 c. thinly sliced strawberries

3/4 c. chopped toasted pecans

1/4 small red onion, thinly sliced

5 oz. feta, crumbled

Instructions

1. In a large bowl, whisk the lemon juice with the mustard. While whisking, slowly pour in the oil until the dressing is combined. Season with salt and pepper.
2. Add spinach, chicken, strawberries, ½ cup pecans, and onion to the bowl with the dressing and toss to combine.

3. Pile salad onto plates and top with the remaining pecans and a generous crumbling of feta.

Cilantro-Lime Cucumber Salad 10%
(with 2 fiber caps)

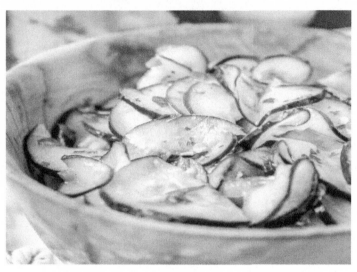

"Click Underlined Colored Word ingredients to buy them!"

Ingredients

1 jalapeno, seeded and finely diced
2 cloves fresh garlic, finely minced
3 tablespoons fresh lime juice
1/4 teaspoon crushed red pepper
1/2 teaspoon salt, or to taste
black pepper to taste
3 tablespoons fresh pressed olive oil
2 cucumbers, very finely sliced (see photos)
4 tablespoons minced cilantro, to taste

Instructions

1. Dice the jalapeno and garlic and add to a medium-sized bowl.
2. Add 3 tablespoons of fresh lime juice, crushed red pepper, salt, and pepper. Use a whisk to incorporate the 3 tablespoons of olive oil. Set aside.

3. Finely slice the cucumbers. Use a mandolin if you have it, but a very sharp knife will do the trick. (See photos below.) Add the cucumbers to the dressing and stir together.
4. Finely mince the cilantro and add it to the bowl. Stir to combine. You can either let it sit in the fridge to marinate for a couple hours, or serve immediately.

Greek Salmon Salad with Tahini Yogurt Dressing 14%(with 2 fiber caps)

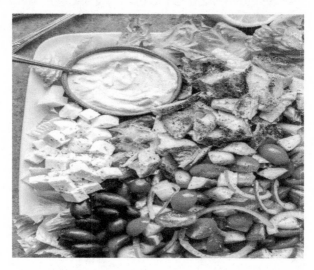

"Click Underlined Colored Word ingredients to buy them!"

Ingredients

4 (4 oz) skin-on wild caught salmon fillets
1/2 teaspoon dried dill
1/2 teaspoon dried oregano
1/4 teaspoon granulated garlic
celtic salt and fresh ground black pepper to taste

For the tahini yogurt dressing
1/2 cup plain (sugar free) Greek yogurt
1 tablespoon tahini
1 1/2 teaspoons fresh pressed olive oil
1 lemon, juiced
1/4 teaspoon ground cumin
1/4 teaspoon dried dill
1/4 teaspoon granulated garlic
1/4 teaspoon coriander
celtic salt and fresh ground black pepper to taste

For the salad

6 cups chopped romaine lettuce
1/3 cup thinly sliced red onion
1/3 cup Kalamata olives
2 ounces feta cheese, cubed
1 cup diced cucumber
1/2 cup cherry tomatoes, halved
1 teaspoon fresh pressed olive oil
1 teaspoon red wine vinegar
1/4 teaspoon dried oregano
1/4 teaspoon dried dill
celtic salt and fresh ground black pepper to taste

Instructions

1. Preheat the grill to medium high heat and oil the grill grates.
2. While the grill heats, combine all of the spices for the salmon and use a mortar and pestle or the palms of your hands to crush them. Sprinkle evenly over the salmon.
3. Place the salmon flesh side down on the grill and cook for 3-5 minutes per side depending on the thickness.
4. Remove from the grill and rest for several minutes before removing the skin and flaking them apart with a fork.
5. In a small bowl combine all of the ingredients for the dressing and whisk together until smooth. Taste for seasoning then refrigerate until ready to serve.
6. In a medium sized bowl whisk together the red wine vinegar, olive oil, oregano, dill, salt and pepper.
7. Add in the diced cucumber, cherry tomatoes and red onion. Toss to combine.
8. On a large platter or in a serving bowl add the romaine lettuce. Top the lettuce with the cucumber mixture, olives, feta and salmon.
9. Serve with the dressing on the side.

InsulThin
Desserts and Treats

Mom's Strawberry Whipped Pie 15%
(with 2 <u>fiber caps</u>)

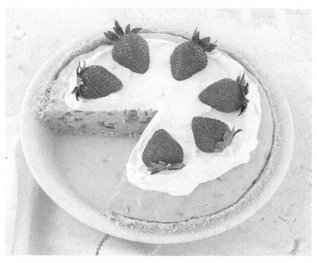

"Click <u>Underlined Colored Word</u> ingredients to buy them!"

This is simply the best tasting extremely lite strawberry pie!
It is from our most considerate and compassionate Mom,

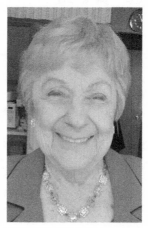

Kathy Grego
(Love you Mom - R.I.P.)

Ingredients

1 pint of fresh organic strawberries
1 package of sugar-free vanilla pudding
1 container of Truwhip
1 premade walnut crust

Instructions

1. Slice up all but 6 large strawberries.
2. Place in a large bowl.
3. Make vanilla pudding with directions provided.
4. Mix pudding with strawberries and Truwhip (all but ¼)
5. Put the premade pecan pie crust.
6. Place in the refrigerator to congeal.
7. Take out and place the ¼ of Truwhip on top of the pie.
8. Gently place the 6 large strawberries on top of the pie
9. And enjoy!

Key Lime Pie 13% (w/ 2 fiber caps)

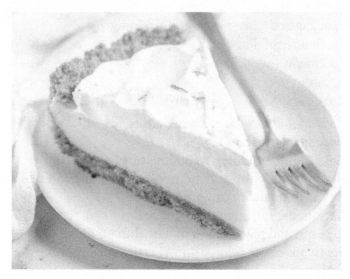

"Click **Underlined Colored Word** ingredients to buy them!"

Ingredients

Crust
Buy a premade pecan crust here.

Filling
2 medium Avocado (very ripe)
12 oz Cream cheese (softened at room temperature or by heating)
4 small Limes
2/3 cup Stevia or Monk fruit powder
1 tsp vanilla

Instructions

1. Line the bottom of a pie pan with parchment paper
2. Buy a premade pecan crust here. Or at Walmart
3. Place the avocado (skin removed), softened cream cheese, powdered sweetener, and vanilla extract into a high power blender or a food processor.
4. Zest the limes using a zester and add the zest to the blender. Squeeze the juice out of all the limes in there as well. Puree

the mixture until smooth, scraping down the sides with a spatula.

5. Pour/spoon the pureed mixture into the crust. Smooth with a spatula or the back of a spoon.

6. Refrigerate for at least, until the pie is firm. Serve with homemade sugar-free whipped cream if desired. Keep refrigerated.

Brownies 13% (w/ 2 fiber caps)

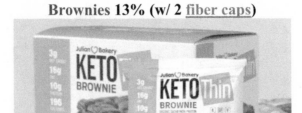

Too tired to make your own brownies . . . Well just Click this InsulThin Brownies . . . and. . . Enjoy!

Chocolate Peanut Butter Pie 14%
(with 2 fiber caps)

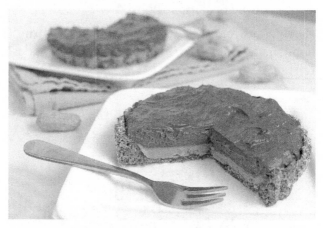

"Click Underlined Colored Word ingredients to buy them!"

Ingredients

Crust buy a premade pecan
Top Layer 1 medium Avocado
4 tbsp. Cocoa powder
1/4 cup Stevia or Monk fruit powder
1/2 tsp. Vanilla Extract
1/2 tsp. Cinnamon
2 tbsp. Heavy Cream
Middle Layer4 tbsp. Santa Cruz Creamy Peanut Butter
2 tbsp. Kerry Butter

Instructions

1. Combine all the top layer ingredients in a small blender until smooth.
2. Melt peanut butter and butter in the microwave or a small pan over the stove until soft.
3. Pour the melted peanut butter layer onto your pie crusts and place in the fridge for about 30 minutes until the top is set.

4. Once the top of the peanut butter layer is set, add the chocolate avocado layer on top and smooth out. Place in the fridge for another 30 minutes and serve!

Marshmallows (helps arthritis/ joint pain)
11% (with 2 fiber caps)

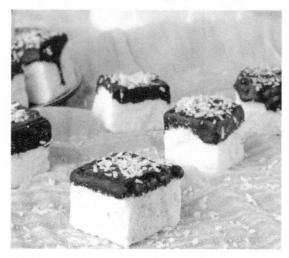

"Click <u>Underlined Colored Word</u> ingredients to buy them!"

Ingredients

3 large egg whites
4 tbsp. gelatin powder
1 tsp **cream of tartar** *or* 1 tsp apple cider vinegar
$^1/_2$ cup <u>Stevia</u> or <u>Monk fruit powder</u>
15-20 drops **liquid Stevia** extract
1 tsp unsweetened **vanilla** extract
$^1/_4$ cup cold <u>Life Ionizer water</u> / Evian water
$^3/_4$ cup boiling <u>Life Ionizer water</u> / Evian water
1 heaping tbsp. <u>coconut flour</u>
pinch of <u>celtic sea salt</u>

Instructions

1. Line an 8 x 8 pan with parchment paper. Sprinkle it with a layer of coconut flour.
2. Place the gelatin into a pot and add $^1/_4$ cup of cold water. The gelatin will become firm in just a couple of minutes.
3. Separate the egg whites from the egg yolks. (watch this <u>video</u>)

4. Using an electric mixer, start beating the egg whites. *Slowly* add the cream of tartar, powdered Stevia/Monk fruit, vanilla and celtic salt.
5. Keep beating for a minute or two until it becomes thick and creates soft peaks.
6. Add the remaining *boiling* water to the pot with the gelatin and stir until dissolved.. Add stevia/monk fruit and combine well.
7. Turn the mixer to medium speed and *very slowly* pour a steady stream of gelatin into the egg whites. After you pour all the gelatin, turn the mixer to high and continue beating until it becomes thick and creamy.
8. Turn off the mixer and quickly transfer the marshmallow cream into the pan lined with parchment paper and sprinkled with fine coconut flour.
9. Spread evenly all over the pan
10. Sprinkle more coconut flour on top and pat level if needed. If you are not using any coating, grease your hands with coconut oil and pat smooth.
11. Place in the fridge for 2-3 hours or overnight until the marshmallow cream is fully set. When done, remove the pan and peel the parchment paper off.
12. Cut into cubes, 4 by 4 to create approx. 40 marshmallows.
13. If you make plain marshmallows with no topping, place on a plate and cover with a towel for a few hours. Then, store them in the fridge in an airtight container to avoid drying.
14. Melt the chocolate in a water bath. Dip a lolly stick into the chocolate and then add the marshmallow. It's best to use a water bath for melting chocolate, especially if it's high in cacao content. Melting chocolate directly could result in burning.
15. Dip each marshmallow into the melted chocolate and keep turning until the chocolate stops dripping.
16. Alternatively, you can skip the lolly stick and just dip the marshmallows in chocolate
17. Sprinkle each marshmallow with shredded coconut and place on parchment paper until the chocolate hardens.
18. Let them dry at room temperature After they dry you can place them in a container lined with paper towel and store them sealed in the fridge.

Optional toppings:

1 dark chocolate choczero bar - 3 tbsp. unsweetened desiccated coconut

Red Velvet Cake 15% (with 2 fiber caps)

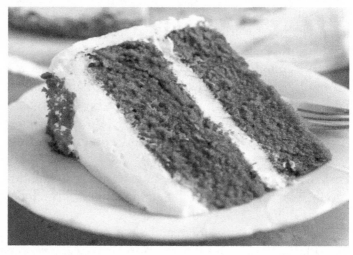

"Click Underlined Colored Word ingredients to buy them!"

Ingredients

Cake Layers
1 1/2 cup Almond Flour
2 cups Confectioners Monk fruit
3/4 cup Kerry Gold Butter salted
3/4 cup Coconut Flour
1 cup Cashew Milk
9 Large Eggs
2 tbsp. Cocoa Powder Unsweetened
2 tsp Vanilla Extract
2 tsp Red Food Coloring
1 tsp Baking Powder
1/2 tsp Xanthan Gum

Cream Cheese Frosting
10 oz Cream Cheese Full Fat
1/2 cup Kerry Gold Butter
1 1/2 cup Confectioners Monk fruit
2 tbsp. Cashew Milk
1 tbsp. Vanilla Extract

Cake Layers

1. Combine coconut flour, almond flour, baking powder and Xanthan gum in a bowl. Stir until incorporated, then set aside.
2. In another bowl, mix together cocoa, monk fruit, cashew milk, and butter. Heat in microwave for 10 seconds at a time until butter is just melted, not extremely hot. (Note: if it's too hot, it will cook the eggs in the next step)
3. Add food coloring, vanilla, and eggs to the warm butter/milk mixture. Mix thoroughly.
4. Slowly pour wet mixture into the dry ingredients. Fold together until well incorporated.
5. Prepare 2 round cake pans spraying the bottom and sides with non stick spray, then line the bottom of the pan with parchment paper. Add a bit more non stick spray on top of the paper as well.
6. Split cake batter between the two prepared pans.
7. Bake 30-35 minutes until a toothpick test comes back clean. The cakes will be fluffy and slightly spongy to the touch.
8. Let the cakes sit in the pans for 10-15 minutes to set up before turning them out onto a cooling rack.
9. Let cool completely before frosting.

Cream Cheese Frosting

1. Cream together room temperature butter and cream cheese until well combined.
2. Slowly add confectioners Monk Fruit sweetener until incorporated.
3. Add Cashew Milk and Vanilla and mix thoroughly. For thicker frosting, add a little less Cashew Milk. For thinner, add just a little more.

Chocolate Chip Cookies 13%
(w/ 2 <u>fiber caps</u>)

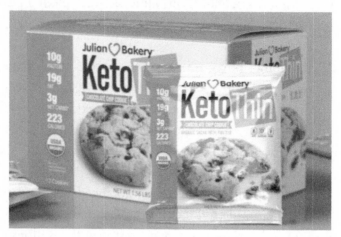

Got in late . . . but still would like a little snack that won't kick you out?
Look no further . .. <u>InsulThin Chocolate Chip Cookies.</u>

Chocolate Peanut Butter Cups 13%
(w/ 2 fiber caps)

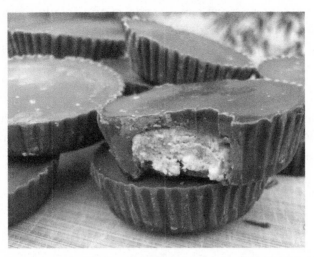

"Click Underlined Colored Word ingredients to buy them!"

Ingredients

For the Chocolate Part

Cocoa Butter: 9 ounces (by weight)
Cocoa Powder: 3 tbsp.
Powdered Monk Fruit: 5 tbsp.
Stevia 5 drops
Pure Vanilla Extract: 1 tsp
Celtic Sea Salt: 1/4 tsp

For the Peanut Butter Filling

Santa Cruz creamy Peanut Butter: 1 cup
Powdered Monk Fruit: 4 tbsp.
Pure Vanilla Extract: 1/2 tsp
Celtic Sea Salt: 1/4 tsp

Instructions

For the chocolate

1. Chop or shred the cocoa butter

2. Melt cocoa butter in microwave for 60-90 seconds, stirring half way through. Make sure it's all melted.
3. Gradually sprinkle cocoa powder and monk fruit into the melted cocoa butter, stirring as you add to prevent clumping.
4. Stir in vanilla and salt.
5. Stir until mixture is smooth.

For the peanut butter

1. Stir all peanut butter ingredients together in a bowl until well incorporated. Mixture will be fairly thick and yummy (**note**: you will want to go ahead and lick the spoon!)

Pecan Pie 15% (w/ 2 <u>fiber caps</u>)

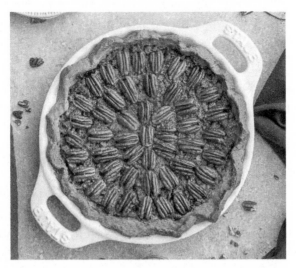

"Click <u>Underlined Colored Word</u> ingredients to buy them!"

For crust: buy a premade <u>pecan crust</u>
For filling
1 cup Kerry butter
1 cup <u>golden monk fruit sweetener</u>
2 tablespoons <u>almond butter</u>
1 cup full fat <u>canned coconut milk</u>
2 teaspoons <u>vanilla extract</u>
1/2 teaspoon <u>Celtic sea salt</u>
3 large eggs , at room temperature
2 cups roughly chopped <u>pecans</u>
1/2 cup half pecans for the topping

Instructions

Make the Filling
1. Preheat the oven to 325°F. Remove the pie pan from the refrigerator and par-bake the crust for 15 minutes or until very light golden brown around the edges. Remove from oven and set aside to cool.
2. Brown Butter - have all the ingredients ready to go as the butter can burn very quickly

3. Heat butter in a large heavy bottomed saucepan over medium heat, whisking constantly. Once the butter starts boiling, continue whisking until you see brown bits starting to form at the bottom of pan as you are whisking. Remove the pan immediately from the heat and turn heat off. Whisk in the golden monk fruit sweetener until combined. Add almond butter, coconut milk, sea salt and vanilla and whisk until smooth.

4. Allow the sauce to cool slightly. Once cool, slowly whisk in the eggs until combined.

5. Stir in the chopped pecans and pour into the par-baked crust.

6. Arrange pecan halves on top to design of your liking.

7. Cover the crust edges with a pie shield or aluminum foil to prevent burning. Bake for 40-45 minutes or until center is nearly set (still a bit jiggly) and crust is deep golden brown.

8. Allow to cool completely at room temperature for at least 1 hour before slicing. If making ahead, wrap and store in the refrigerator for up to 2 days.

9. Start by melting butter in a heavy duty pot over medium heat. Swirl the pot occasionally to prevent burning.

10. The butter will begin to foam and the color will go from lemony-yellow to golden-tan to, finally, a toasty-brown. Once you smell that nutty aroma, take the pan off the heat and transfer the browned butter into a heat-proof bowl to cool.

11. You want to make sure the caramel filling is cool enough to not scramble the egg but not completely cool that it will start to solidify.

12. You'll whisk in the monk fruit sweetener, followed by the full fat canned coconut milk, almond butter, vanilla extract and sea salt.

13. When the sauce is cool enough, beat in the eggs until smooth then stir in the chopped pecans.

14. Transfer the filling to the par-baked crust.

15. Top with pecans in desired pattern then bake in preheated oven at 325 F for 40-50 minutes or until the filling has set

16. You can cover the crust with aluminum foil to prevent the crust from browning too much.
17. This dairy free pecan pie filling bakes up nice, gooey and rich with a balanced sweetness.
18. This sugar free pecan pie recipe makes the perfect dessert.

Pecan Pie Cheesecake 15% (w/ 2 fiber caps)

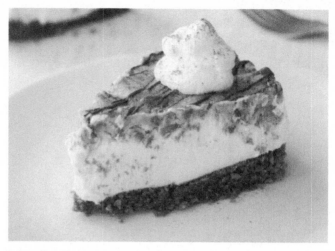

"Click <u>Underlined Colored Word</u> ingredients to buy them!"

Ingredients

Pecan/Walnut **Crust**
Buy it premade at Walmart

Cheesecake Layer
16 oz Cream Cheese

1 cup *Monk fruit powder*, or Stevia

2/3 cup Heavy Whipping Cream

2 tsp Vanilla Extract

Caramel Layer
5 tbsp. Butter; divided

1/2 cup *Monk fruit powder*, or Stevia

2 tbsp. Heavy Whipping Cream

1/2 tsp Vanilla Extract

1 1/2 cup Chopped Pecans

Instructions

Cheesecake Layer

1. In a large mixing bowl, place softened cream cheese and beat for 3 minutes until completely smooth. Add Stevia/Monk fruit and beat for an additional 3 minutes.
2. Add heavy whipping cream and vanilla. Whip for 5-7 minutes or until mixture is completely smooth.
3. Pour mixture onto cooled (or mostly cooled) crust and spread evenly. Place in the freezer while you prepare the final layer.

Caramel Pecan Layer

1. In a skillet or saucepan over medium-low heat add 4 tbsp. butter. Once butter is almost completely melted add stevia / monk fruit.. Stir frequently with rubber spatula and watch closely as it turns golden brown.
2. Once it is light or golden brown, add heavy cream and pecans. Continue gentle stirring frequently until dark golden brown. Turn off heat and add final tablespoon of butter. Let the mixture cool for 10 minutes.
3. Mixture should still be very hot but cooled from the near boiling point. Remove cheesecake from the freezer and pour caramel pecan mixture over top, using rubber spatula to even layer. Try to make sure all pecan pieces are flat and level with caramel for best results. You may need to press them down gently or gently move the pan back and forth to level.
4. Then place in premade crust.
5. Place in the fridge overnight to completely cool. If the mixture is not completely cool when cut into, the top layer will not stay together.
6. Place in the freezer for 2-3 hours before you're going to eat it. Freezing it will firm up the cheesecake layer and allow you to slice through the top layer without it cracking.

Chewy Double Chocolate Chip Cookies 15% (w/ 2 fiber caps)

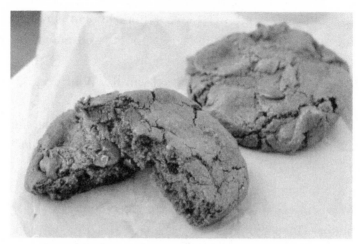

"Click Underlined Colored Word ingredients to buy them!"

Ingredients

1 cup natural creamy almond butter
2/3 cup stevia / monk fruit powder
2 tablespoons unsweetened cocoa powder
2 tablespoons Santa Cruz Creamy peanut butter
2 large eggs
1 tablespoon melted salted Kerry butter
2 tablespoons Life ionizer water / Evian water
1 1/2 teaspoons vanilla extract
1 teaspoon baking soda
1/4 cup choczero baking chips

Instructions

1. Preheat the oven to 350°F. Line a rimmed baking sheet with a silicone baking mat or parchment paper.
2. In a large mixing bowl, combine the almond butter, stevia/monk fruit, cocoa powder, peanut butter powder, eggs, butter, water, vanilla extract, and baking soda. Using an electric hand mixer, mix until all ingredients are well combined. It will be a very thick dough. Fold in the chocolate chips.

3. Form the cookie dough into 1 1/2 inch to 2 inch balls.
4. Place the cookie dough balls on the prepared baking sheet. Bake for 8 to 11 minutes (begin checking on them at 8 minutes).
5. Remove the baking sheet from the oven and place on a cooling rack to allow the cookies to cool before eating

Chocolate Chip Cookies 15% (w/ 2 <u>fiber caps</u>)

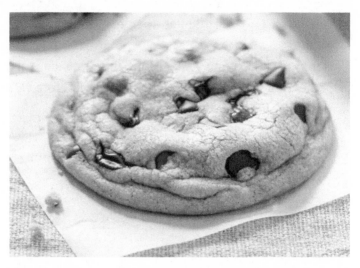

"Click <u>Underlined Colored Word</u> ingredients to buy them!"

Ingredients

2 large eggs
1/2 c. (1 stick) melted <u>Kerry butter</u>
2 tbsp. <u>heavy cream</u>
2 tsp. pure <u>vanilla extract</u>
2 3/4 c. <u>almond flour</u>
1/4 tsp. <u>Celtic salt</u>
1 c. <u>Stevia/Monk Fruit powder</u>
3/4 c. <u>Choczero dark chocolate chips</u>
<u>Cooking spray</u>

DIRECTIONS

1. Preheat the oven to 350°. In a large bowl, whisk the egg with the butter, heavy cream, and vanilla. Stir in the almond flour, salt, and powdered sugar.
2. Fold the chocolate chips into the cookie batter. Form the batter into 1" balls and arrange 3" apart on parchment lined baking sheets. Flatten the balls with the bottom of a glass that has been lightly greased with cooking spray.
3. Bake until the cookies are golden, about 17 to 19 minutes.

Pumpkin Pie 13% (w/ 2 <u>fiber caps</u>)

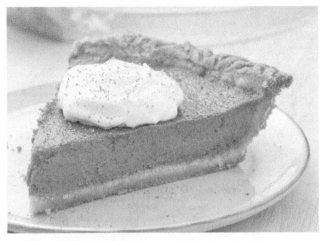

"Click <u>Underlined Colored Word</u> ingredients to buy them!"

Ingredients

For The Crust- Go <u>here</u>

For The Filling
1 (15-oz.) can organic pumpkin puree
1 c. heavy cream
1/2 c. <u>Stevia</u> / <u>Monk fruit powder</u>
3 large eggs, beaten
1 tsp. <u>ground cinnamon</u>
1/2 tsp. <u>ground ginger</u>
1/4 tsp. <u>ground nutmeg</u>
1/4 tsp. <u>ground cloves</u>

Instructions

1. In a large bowl, whisk together pumpkin, cream, brown sugar, eggs, spices, and vanilla until smooth. Pour pumpkin mixture into pre-baked crust.
2. Bake at 350 until filling is slightly jiggly in the middle and crust is golden, 45 to 50 minutes.
3. Turn off oven and prop door open. Let pie cool in oven for 1 hour, then refrigerate until ready to serve.
4. Serve with True whipped cream.

Peanut Butter Fat Bombs 15% (w/ 2 <u>fiber caps</u>)

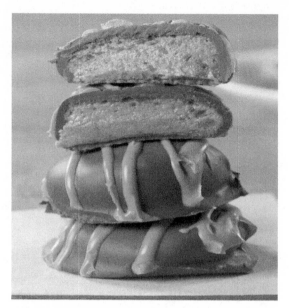

"Click <u>Underlined Colored Word</u> ingredients to buy them!"

Ingredients

1 1/2 c. smooth <u>Santa Cruz creamy peanut butter</u>, melted
1 c. coconut flour fine
1/2 c. <u>Stevia</u> / <u>Monk fruit powder</u>
1 tsp. pure <u>vanilla extract</u>
Pinch <u>celtic sea salt</u>
2 c. <u>ChocZero dark chocolate baking chips</u>
1 tbsp. <u>Dr. Bronner's coconut oil</u>

Instructions

1. In a medium bowl, combine peanut butter, coconut flour, coconut sugar, vanilla, and salt. Stir until smooth.
2. Line a baking sheet with parchment paper. Using a small cookie scoop, form mixture into rounds then press down lightly to flatten slightly and place on baking sheet. Freeze until firm, about 1 hour.
3. In a medium bowl, whisk together melted chocolate and coconut oil.

4. Using a fork, dip peanut butter rounds in chocolate until fully coated then return to baking sheet. Drizzle with more peanut butter then freeze until chocolate sets, about 10 minutes.

5. Serve cold. Store any leftovers in the freezer.

Avocado Brownies 15% (w/ 2 <u>fiber caps</u>)

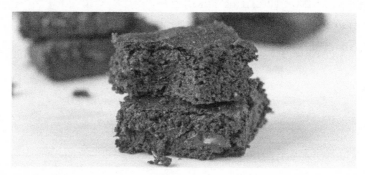

"Click <u>Underlined Colored Word</u> ingredients to buy them!"

Ingredients

4 large eggs
2 ripe avocados
1/2 c. (1 stick) melted <u>Kerry butter</u>
6 tbsp. <u>Santa Cruz creamy peanut butter</u>
2 tsp. <u>baking soda</u>
1 c. <u>Stevia</u> / <u>Monk fruit powder</u>
2/3 c. unsweetened <u>cocoa powder</u>
2 tsp. pure <u>vanilla extract</u>
1/2 tsp. <u>Celtic sea salt</u>

Instructions

1. Preheat the oven to 350° and line an 8"-x-8" square pan with parchment paper. In a blender or food processor, combine all ingredients except flaky sea salt and blend until smooth.
2. Transfer batter to prepared baking pan and smooth top with a spatula. Top with flaky sea salt, if using.
3. Bake until brownies are soft but not at all wet to the touch, 25 to 30 minutes.
4. Let cool 25 to 30 minutes before slicing and serving.

Coconut Crack Bars 13% (w/ 2 <u>fiber caps</u>)

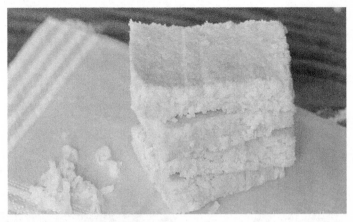

"Click <u>Underlined Colored Word</u> ingredients to buy them!"

Ingredients

3 cups <u>Shredded unsweetened coconut flakes</u>
1 cup <u>coconut oil,</u> melted
¼ cup <u>Liquid Stevia</u> / <u>Monk fruit</u>

Instructions

1. Line an 8 x 8-inch pan or 8 x 10-inch pan with parchment paper and set aside. Alternatively, you can use a loaf pan.
2. In a large mixing bowl, add your shredded unsweetened coconut. Add your melted coconut oil and Stevia/monk fruit and mix until a thick batter remains. If it is too crumbly, add a little extra syrup or a tiny bit of water.
3. Pour the coconut crack bar mixture into the lined pan. Lightly wet your hands and press firmly into place. Refrigerate or freeze until firm. Cut into bars and enjoy!

Lemon Pound Cake 15% (w/ 2 <u>fiber caps</u>)

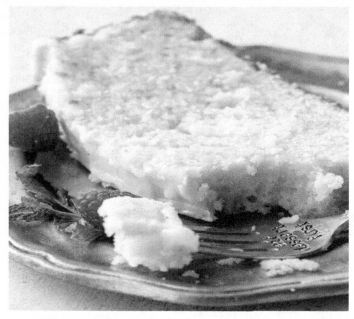

"Click <u>Underlined Colored Word</u> ingredients to buy them!"

Ingredients

5 eggs - at room temperature
3/4 cup <u>Stevia / Monk fruit powder</u>
1/2 cup melted <u>coconut oil</u>
2 cups <u>fine almond flour</u>
1/4 cup <u>fine coconut flour</u>
1 tablespoon <u>aluminum free baking powder</u>
1/4 cup organic lemon juice

Lemon Glazing
1 cup <u>powdered Stevia/Monk fruit powder</u>
2 tablespoon organic lemon juice

Instructions

For the Cake
1. Preheat the oven to 350F Line a loaf pan 9 inches x 5 inches with a piece of parchment paper. Slightly oil the paper to make sure the pound cake doesn't stick to the pan. Set aside.

2. In a medium mixing bowl, whisk together eggs, sugar free crystal sweetener, melted coconut oil (or butter) and lemon juice. Make sure that your coconut oil is not burning hot or it will 'cook' the eggs and create lumps. All your ingredients must be roughly at same temperature, think room temperature especially the eggs and lemon juice. Cold ingredients, just out of the fridge will solidify the coconut oil creating oil lumps. Otherwise use melted butter to prevent this from happening. Set aside.

3. In a different large mixing bowl, whisk together the almond flour, coconut flour and baking powder. Stir to evenly combine the flours.

4. Pour the liquid ingredients onto the dry ingredients.

5. Stir all the ingredients together with a baking spoon until it forms a consistent cake batter with no lumps. Combine for at least 2 minutes to make sure the coconut flour fiber absorbs the moisture.

6. Transfer the cake batter onto the loaf pan. Make sure you are using the same loaf pan size or it will impact your baking time.

7. Place the loaf pan in the center of your oven and bake at 350F, fan-forced mode if you can for 15 minutes. After 15 minutes decrease the temperature to 320F and cover the loaf pan with a loose piece of foil. This will avoid the top to burn and the middle to bake slowly. Keep baking for 45- 60 minutes in total, or until a toothpick inserted in the center of the pound cake comes out with little to no crumbs on it.

8. Cool for 10 minutes in the loaf pan, then lift out the pound cake from the pan using the parchment paper.

9. Transfer to a cooling rack to cool completely. It is a thick cake and it usually takes 3 hours to fully cool. Be patient and add the lemon glazing on the cake when it reaches room temperature, not before!

For the Lemon Glazing

1. To make the lemon glazing, whisk together the sugar free powdered Stevia/Monk fruit with lemon juice until no lumps remain. If needed add more lemon juice to get a thinner glazing or more powdered sweetener to get a thicker glazing.

2. Drizzle consistency over the cooled pound cake.

3. You can place the cake a few minutes in the freezer to set the glazing if too runny.

4. Store your cake in the pantry on a cake box for up to 3 or 4 days. Slice before serving to keep the cake moist.

Peanut Butter Cookies 15% (w/ 2 <u>fiber caps</u>)

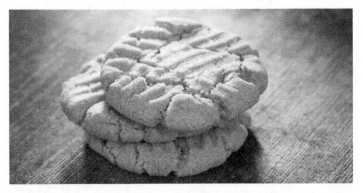

"Click <u>Underlined Colored Word</u> ingredients to buy them!"

Ingredients

½ C <u>Stevia</u> / <u>Monk fruit power</u>
1 egg
1/2 teaspoon **<u>vanilla extract</u>**
225 g **<u>Santa Cruz creamy peanut butter</u>**
1/4 teaspoon <u>celtic sea salt</u>

Instructions

1. Preheat the oven to 350°F and line a baking tray with parchment paper or a baking mat.
2. Add the sweetener, and egg to a medium bowl and beat with an electric mixer (or whisk!) until light and fluffy, about 3 minutes.
3. Mix in the vanilla extract, followed by the peanut butter.
4. Scoop out the cookie dough, form into rounds and press down with a fork. Place in a prepared tray and freeze for 15 minutes prior to baking.
5. Bake for 12-14 minutes, until lightly golden and set.
6. Allow to cool completely before digging and store in an airtight container for 3-4 days or in the freezer for up to 3 months.

Peanut Butter Chocolate Chip Cookies
15% (w/ 2 fiber caps)

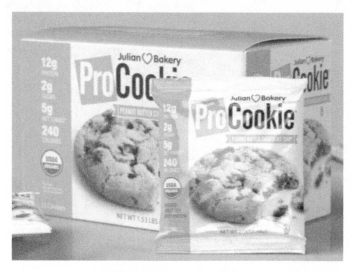

Need we say more?
Click Here . . .and Smile!

Strawberry Shortcake 13% (w/ 2 <u>fiber caps</u>)

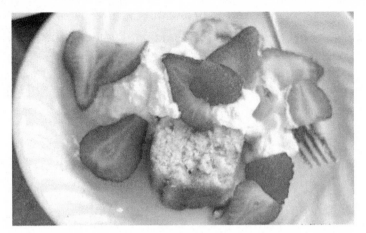

"Click <u>Underlined Colored Word</u> ingredients to buy them!"

Ingredients

4 tbsp. <u>Kerry butter</u> softened
1/2 cup <u>Stevia</u> / <u>Monk fruit powder</u>
4 eggs
1 tsp <u>vanilla liquid</u>
1/4 cup sour cream
1 1/4 cup <u>fine almond flour</u>
1/4 cup <u>fine coconut flour</u>
1/4 cup <u>ground fine flax seed</u>
1 tsp <u>baking powder</u>
1/4 tsp <u>celtic sea salt</u>
3/4 cup organic strawberries chopped

Whipped Cream

1 pint <u>heavy cream</u>
2 tbsp. <u>Stevia</u> / <u>Monk fruit powder</u>

Instructions

1. Preheat the oven to 350. Grease a loaf pan liberally with butter.
2. In a bowl with an electric mixer cream the butter and gently sweet until light and fluffy. Add the sour cream and vanilla and beat until combined. Add the eggs one at a time, mixing after each.

3. Stir in the flours, baking powder, and salt until thoroughly combined. Fold in the strawberries. Pour into loaf pan and spread evenly.
4. Bake at 350 for 45-60 min until golden, firm to the touch, and no longer jiggly.
5. Meanwhile, whip the cream. Once peaks form add the sweetener. Refrigerate until ready to serve. Slice the cake and serve with whipped cream and extra organic regenerative berries.

Enlightened Ice Cream 13% (w/ 2 fiber caps)

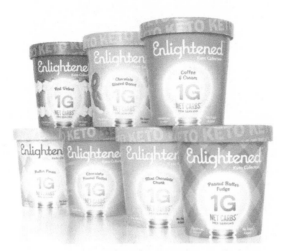

Over 10 different and delicious flavors!

Only 1 - 3 grams of Carbs! Buy at Publix and Here

Rebel Ice Cream 15% (w/ 2 <u>fiber caps</u>)

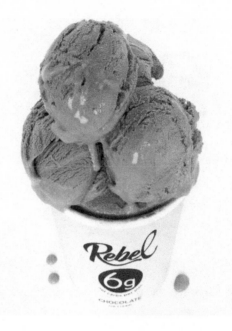

Yes That's right delicious low carb ice-cream no sugar - all tasty!

14 different succulent flavors!

Available at Publix and at <u>here</u>

Buff Bake Fuel Bar 12%

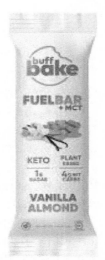

High fat, low carb
No sugar alcohols
Snack!
You can get them here

Stevia Dent Sugar-Free Gum

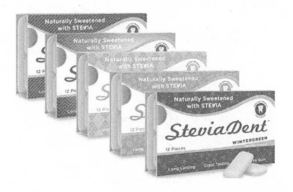

Our stevia-sweetened gum fulfills your cravings with fewer calories, and without harming your teeth. The stable gum base keeps its minty wintergreen flavor, allowing you to enjoy our chewing gum as long as you want. It comes in 5 breath freshening flavors: cinnamon, wintergreen, peppermint, spearmint and fruit.
You can buy it here.

ChocZero 9% (w/ 2 fiber caps)

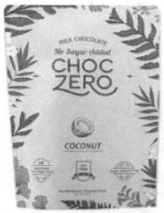

Only the best tasting chocolate bars on the planet!
12 different mouth-watering flavors
And Maple Syrups
And Chocolate nibs for baking

Sweetened only with Monk fruit!
Get them here

ChocZero Peanut Butter Cups 13%
(w/ 2 <u>fiber caps</u>)

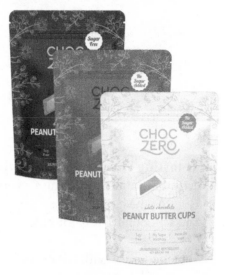

These are Dr. Grego's favorite go to <u>snacks</u>!
They are sweetened with Monk Fruit.
They have No Sugar Alcohols.

Appetizers / Dips

**Try These Delicious
<u>Crackers</u> with Your Dips**

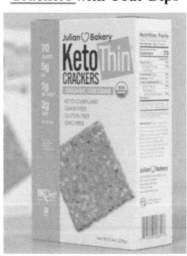

Queso Dip In A Crock Pot 13%
(with 2 fiber caps)

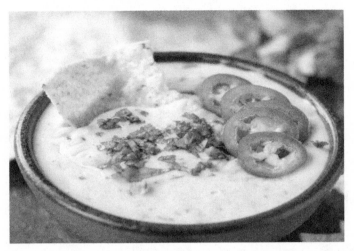

"Click Underlined Colored Word ingredients to buy them!"

Ingredients

8 oz Cream cheese (cut into cubes)
12 oz Salsa
1 cup Monterey jack cheese
Cilantro fresh
Jalapenos sliced thin
Keto Chips

Instructions

1. Mix all ingredients together in a slow cooker. Cook for 2 1/2 hours on low, stirring and whisking every 30 minutes to get rid of any lumps.
2. Optional: If you want even smoother dip, you can puree it in a blender at the end. Return to the slow cooker on the Warm setting to keep the dip warm.
3. Garnish with cilantro and Jalapenos . . .
4. Dip with delicious low carb high fat Keto Chips . . . . Enjoy!!!

Caramelized French Onion Dip 12%
(with 2 fiber caps)

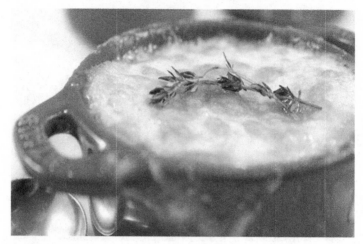

"Click <u>Underlined Colored Word</u> ingredients to buy them!"

Ingredients

2 tbsp. <u>Kerry Salted butter</u>
2 large Vidalia or Sweet Onions
1/4 cup Bone broth
4 cloves Garlic (minced)
2 cups Sour Cream
4 oz Cream cheese (softened)
1/4 tsp liquid Stevia/Monk fruit
2 tbsp. Fresh thyme
1/2 tsp <u>Celtic sea salt</u>

Instructions

1. Heat the butter in a large sauté pan over medium heat. Add the onions and 2 tablespoons of bone broth. Sauté for 30 min, adding another 2 more tablespoons of broth after the first 10-15 minutes to keep the onions hydrated, and continue to sauté until browned and caramelized. Reduce heat if they start to brown too much.

2. Make a well in the center of the pan. Add the minced garlic and sauté for about a minute. Once the garlic is fragrant and

starting to brown, stir into the onions. Set the pan aside to cool to room temperature.

3. Meanwhile, in a medium bowl, stir together the sour cream, softened cream cheese, molasses, fresh thyme, and sea salt, until smooth.

4. Once the caramelized onions have cooled, stir them into the bowl. Add more salt to taste if desired. If you want a firmer dip, chill for at least 30 min.

5. TIP: If you would like a firmer dip, chill for 30 minutes

Cucumber Guacamole Appetizer 12%
(with <u>2 fiber caps</u>)

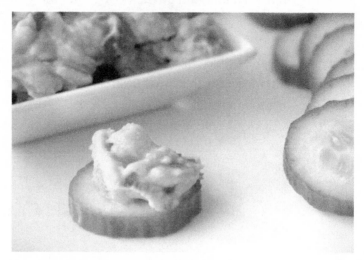

"Click <u>Underlined Colored Word</u> ingredients to buy them!"

Ingredients

1 large European cucumber
1 cup guacamole purchased or made with premix packet and
1 medium avocado
Chile powder for sprinkling on top

Instructions

1. Wash and dry the outside of the cucumber if needed. Peel off strips of the skin if you like that look, or don't like the taste of the skin.
2. Cut the cucumber into slices that are about 5/8 inch thick, discarding the ends.
3. Put the guacamole into a small Ziploc bag; then carefully snip off the corner of the bag.
4. Lay cucumber pieces out on a serving dish
5. Carefully squeeze out enough guacamole to fill the center of each piece of cucumber.
6. Sprinkle each one with the tiniest pinch of chile powder.

Note:
You can use instant Guacamole package or a purchased guacamole for this recipe.

Thai Roasted Cauliflower w/Spicy Peanut Dipping Sauce 8%(with 2 fiber caps)

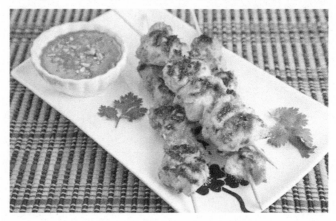

"Click Underlined Colored Word ingredients to buy them!"

Ingredients

Dipping Sauce

1/2 cup warm Life Ionizer water / Evian water

1/4 cup **Santa Cruz chunky peanut butter**

1 tbsp. **apple cider vinegar**

2 tsp **coconut aminos**

1 clove garlic chopped

1/2 tsp red pepper flakes

1/2 tsp ground ginger

Roasted Cauliflower

1 tsp coriander

1/2 tsp cumin

1/2 tsp garlic powder

1/4 tsp ginger

1/4 tsp cayenne

1 large head cauliflower cut into small florets

1/4 cup melted coconut oil

Lime wedges for garnish

1 small bunch of fresh cilantro to garnish
Squire sticks

Instructions

Dipping Sauce

1. Combine Kagin/Evian water, peanut butter, vinegar, aminos or soy sauce, garlic, pepper flakes and ginger in a blender. Blend until almost smooth.

Cauliflower

1. Preheat oven to 400F.
2. In a small bowl, combine coriander, cumin, garlic powder, ginger, and cayenne. Set aside.
3. In a large bowl, toss cauliflower florets with coconut oil. Add spice mixture and toss to coat.
4. Slide cauliflower onto sticks and place on a large baking sheet and roast 15 to 20 minutes, or until tender and beginning to brown.
5. Serve with lime wedges and peanut dipping sauce on the side.

Sriracha Deviled Eggs 13%(with <u>2 fiber caps</u>)

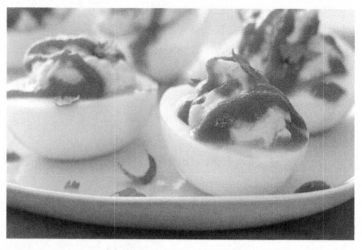

"Click <u>Underlined Colored Word</u> ingredients to buy them!"

Ingredients

7 eggs
3 T mayo
1 1/2 tsp Boars head honey mustard
1-2 tsp. Sriracha sauce
1/2 tsp. <u>Celtic sea salt</u>
1 small bunch of fresh cilantro

Instructions

1. Boil eggs until hardened..
2. After eggs have cooled, running them under ice water will help, peel carefully and cut in half. Carefully remove the yolk from each egg half.
3. Put yolks in a small bowl and arrange the 12 best white egg halves on a tray
4. Mash yolks thoroughly with a fork, then mix in the mayo, mustard, Sriracha, and salt.
5. Taste to see if you want more Sriracha.
6. Use a rubber scraper to put the egg yolk mixture into a small plastic bag, then cut off one corner and squeeze the yolk

mixture out to fill the egg white halves. (I usually use a fork after to smooth out the filling.)

7. Pull cilantro apart and . . . .
8. Sprinkle each egg with a few pieces of cilantro and drizzle Sriracha on top
9. serve.
10. These will definitely keep in the refrigerator for a day or two, so you might want to double the recipe.

Spiced Bacon Deviled Eggs 13%
(with 2 fiber caps)

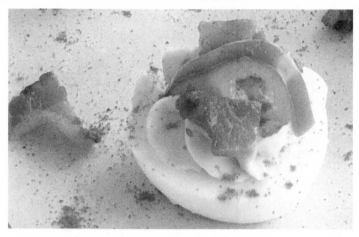

"Click <u>Underlined Colored Word</u> ingredients to buy them!"

Ingredients

5 large hard boiled eggs

¼ cup mayonnaise

2 slices bacon

1 tablespoon rendered bacon fat

1 teaspoon Dijon mustard

¼ teaspoon cayenne pepper

½ teaspoon rosemary

Instructions

1. Slice up your bacon into thin slices and add them to a pan on medium heat.

2. Take out your bacon, keeping as much of the drippings in the pan as possible. Rest your bacon on paper towels to cool off and get extra crispy.

3. Cut your hard-boiled eggs in half. Scoop out all of the yolks with a spoon and add them to a bowl.

4. Add your mayonnaise, Dijon mustard, cayenne pepper, bacon fat, and HALF of 1/4 tsp. rosemary. The rest will be used to garnish.

5. Add some small pieces of bacon to the bottom of the eggs, where the yolk used to be.
6. Mix all of your ingredients together in your bowl. Add the mixture to a piping bag or Ziploc with a corner cut off.
7. Pipe your mixture on the top of the eggs. Add bacon and the rest of the rosemary for garnish.

BONUS CHAPTER

What do I eat if I am at a Restaurant?

We get this question a lot and here are our best solutions:
#1 RULE when eating out at any restaurant is . . . .

Ask the waiter: *"Do You Have Real Butter?"* - if the answer is Yes . .
Would you please melt some real butter in a small bowl for me?

And then dip all your veggies and keto food in butter and voila! You have a great tasting and high fat food - that will keep your % Insulin Rise to < 15%.

#2 RULE when eating out at any restaurant is . . .

Carry a bottle of Liquid Stevia with you *at all times* so you can . .

Order Unsweetened Tea - Unsweetened Coffee - Unsweetened Lemonade etc. and just add a few drops of . . .

Liquid Stevia to those unsweetened drinks and you are good to go!

#3 RULE when eating out at any restaurant is . . .

is to have a baggie of **Fiber Caps** in your pocket.
So you can take 2 or 3 to bring down the Insulin Rise of any food or drink.

HINT: If you are ever unsure about a food or drink Insulin Rise potential . .
Use this link to Your **INSULIN CALCULATOR** and check it.

Burger King

They came out with the Impossible Whopper, which is vegan, and is doable without the bread of course. DON'T EAT THIS - IT IS MADE OUT OF GMO SOY.

Any burger (with or without bacon) - and of course no bun.
Any Salad . Use balsamic or oil and vinegar dressing.

McDonald's - Wendy's - Chick Fil A - Panera Bread

Get a sandwich without the bun - have them put it in a bowl with salad and either balsamic vinegar or oil and vinegar dressing.

Denny's - has the delicious beyond meat burger. With a big salad of your choice.

Hardies - has the Beyond Meat Sausage. No bun.

Taco Bell - Power Menu Bowl - Veggie - Chicken or Beef and just ask them to hold the beans and add extra guac.

5 Guys - Cook Out - Arby's - Subway - In and Out Burger - Whataburger

Ask for a bowl with chicken or beef and lettuce and then use their sides to make a salad to your taste:

- Mayo
- Lettuce
- Pickles
- Tomatoes
- Grilled Onions
- Grilled Mushrooms
- Ketchup
- Mustard
- Relish
- Onions
- Jalapeño Peppers
- Green Peppers
- Bar-B-Que Sauce
- Hot Sauce

Pizza Hut - Domino's - Little Caesars - Papa John's - CiCi's - Mellow Mushroom

This is a little exception, you can order a pizza (cheese) with any of the veggie toppings, just no crust.
Have them cook all the ingredients and then put them in a bowl instead of on a crust.

Chipotle - Moe's

This is easy - order a bowl with chicken beef or tofu and veggies, spinach and guac and salsa.

Bojangles - Steak N Shake - Churches - Captain D's - Zaxby's

Get the chicken or fish without the bread. Have them fix it in a bowl instead.
Coleslaw from Churches and Captain D's. And side salads/Cobb salad with all the veggies they offer and vinegar and oil dressing from the rest on this list.

Indian Food
My (dr. Grego) personal favorite restaurant food. **Baingan Bharta** which is my personal favorite and an eggplant dish. Wonderfully exotic and tasty! Some of the best vegan Indian InsulThin dishes are as follows:

1 **Seitan Vindaloo**- no potatoes. In this recipe, meaty seitan is smothered in a spicy and tangy tomato-based curry. This traditional Indian dish is flavorful, affordable, and easy to make. Enjoy wafting in the delicious curry aroma of this fragrant dish!

2 **Punjabi Chana Masala** - substitute eggplant for the chickpeas. This is super special. No garlic/tomatoes. Cooked with tamarind, it is one of those curries which will definitely stand out in the lot. This recipe has been passed over for generations and I am sure it will for many more. I have eaten a fair share of curries but nothing this unique.

3 **Palak 'Paneer'**- Tofu stands in for dairy cheese to make the paneer in Nikki and Zuzana's Palak "Paneer" made with spinach. It has just the right amount of spices to make it incredibly flavorful. Make sure you take your milk pill.

4 **Paneer' Tikka Masala** - Tikka masala is a popular North Indian recipe usually made with chicken. In Pavithra Kannan's "Paneer" Tikka Masala, tofu is cooked in spices for an incredible vegan version of this authentic dish.

5 **South Indian-Style Kurma** - Kurma is a South Indian curry dish. Charanya Ramakrishnan's recipe for South Indian Kurma has a variety of vegetables flavored with fennel, cumin, and poppy seeds, cashews and shredded coconut for an amazing meal

Thai Cuisine

The great thing about Thai is that most of their curry's have a base made with coconut milk! So with that in mind, here is a list of options:
Massaman Curry with chicken, beef or veggies - NO potatoes - ADD avocado.* My Favorite!
Panang Curry with chicken, beef or veggies - NO potatoes - ADD avocado.
Red Curry with chicken, beef or veggies - NO potatoes - ADD avocado.
Green Curry with chicken beef or veggies - NO potatoes - ADD avocado.
Coconut soup
Ginger Salad

American Food

Ah yes, hamburgers and hot dogs, french fries and diet cokes! Well just take off the buns and change the french fries for salads. As for the diet cokes - get unsweetened tea or unsweetened lemonade and add your stevia drops.

Mexican Food

One of our favorites is so many good InsulThin choices . . . starting with guacamole! Then you can have any of the burritos without the wraps of course. And you can order veggie fajitas with the sour cream and pico de gallo. Don't forget to top them off with lots of salsa!

Italian Food

Well this is a bit more challenging . . . carbs, carbs, and more carbs!
So you are looking at a nice big antipasto salad without the pasta.
All the oil and vinegar dressing and steamed veggies you can handle.

Soul Food

Well now here in the south we have a lot of Soul Food restaurants and they have a good amount of InsulThin choices. Such as a veggie chicken or beef plate made with coleslaw, collards, mustard greens, turnip tops, dandelions and rhubarb! So good you want to reach up and slap your Mama! (southern sayin' lol)

Chinese Food

Tofu chicken or beef steamed and then baked for extra crispness with all the broccoli, water chestnuts, string beans, and cabbage you can eat! Any of the brown sauces, soy sauce, and yellow mustard you can handle

The Sweet Cycle (of Death) [video tutorial 35]

The below diagram shows how we spiral down from disabling disease to a tortuous death. When we eat the standard American diet or S.A.D.

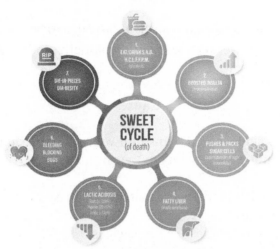

Starting at **#1** = Your eating and drinking from the standard American diet

(S.A.D) or high carb (sugar) low fat, ultra processed food like substances,
stored in plastic and then microwaved. Which turns out …

Causes

#2 Boosted or elevated levels of your insulin (hyperinsulinemia) which…

Causes

#3 Your cells to reach their maximum capacity with sugar (supersaturation) which…

Causes

#4 Your insulin to be ineffective = insulin resistance = fatty liver disease which…

Causes

#5 Metabolic Dx (Lactic acidosis) = your cells become dysfunctional/dis-eased by being
  a) Toxic = lowering your voltage less than -25mV (normal cell charge)
  b) Hypoxic = lowering your 02 to less than 97% oxygen (Sp02)
  c) Acidic = lowering your pH (interstitially) to less than 7 pH which...

Causes

#6 **Bleeding** = acidic blood burns thru your arteries examples: strokes, blindness (diabetic retinopathy), abdominal aneurysms, etc.
  Blocking = toxic blood lowers voltage and makes white fat (instead of brown fat) which is inflammation (mucous) which makes chronic diseases such as infections (virus cytokine storm), heart disease, asthma, cancer, high blood pressure and **chronic pain**.
  Bugs = hypoxic (low 02) blood wakes up bugs (bacteria, fungus, virus, mold, parasites and even cancer) because they are are all anaerobic vectors (they live without 02)

Causes

#7 **You to die - in - pieces** all because you ate and drank from the . . .

"Ultra Processed Standard American Diet"
So, the diagram below shows how to fix all that . .

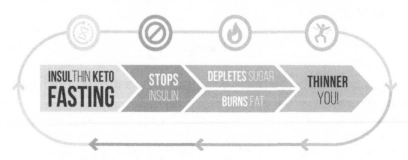

"Knowledge without Action is just entertainment!"
-Dr. Grego

RESOURCES
Must haves when doing InsulThin Diet

"Nothing in life has any meaning until or unless thinking makes it
so . . .
so, who's in charge of your thinking?"
-Tony Robbins

1 Free **"Lazy Way to Lose Weight"** Webinar Click <u>HERE</u>

2 TikTok - <u>TikTok KetoDoc</u>

3 YouTube - *Dr. Grego Keto Doc*

4 <u>Rapid Ketosis</u> - only ketone supplement with fat emulsifiers.
Also with Apple Cider Vinegar and L-Carnitine. A super easy way to get into ketosis and if you make a mistake
by eating to many carbs . . . just 2 capsules and voila! Your back in keto.

5 <u>The Olive Oil Club</u> - I will be honest and say . . when my friend Big Steve asked . . no, pleaded with me to try this "special" olive oil . . .I thought,
Ok. . . No . . way this is any different than any other olive oil. Well 2 months later I tried it . . .and. . . WOW . . .What a difference. . . night and day!
You will look for reasons to put this fresh olive oil on your food!

6 <u>Food Fix Book</u> - Help to transform the planet in crisis with this indispensable guide to healthy, ethical, and economically sustainable food from #1 New York Times bestselling author Mark Hyman, MD

7 Food Policy Action Group - Food Policy Action was established in 2012 through a collaboration of national food policy leaders in order to hold legislators accountable on votes that have an effect on food and farming. Our goal is to change the national dialogue on food policy by educating the public on how elected officials are voting on these issues. Through education and the National Food Policy Scorecard, more people will be armed with the information they need to vote with their forks and elect more food policy leaders across the country.

8 Best Keto Wines - At Dry Farm Wines, we source wines according to our uncompromising criteria of farming and purity. We vet every grower, taste every wine, and ensure every wine is lab tested through an independent enologist. Every bottle in our collection is:
Organic/Biodynamic   Sugar Free(<1g/L)   Free of Toxic Additives

9 Brain Tap - A fantastic Neuro Hack for your brain to de-stress and get into keto. This technology is safe and super effective in regulating neurotransmitters like dopamine and serotonin (feel good hormones). And down regulating stressors like cortisol. This is great for sleep aid and emotional eating disorders.

10 Julian Bakery - All your InsulThin Diet favorite bakery goods . . .like granola cereal, baked breads, crackers, cookies and more!

11 Digestive enzymes
This blend helps your body to digest and assimilate all nutrients necessary for proper, healthy, and permanent weight loss and healing. Each time you use it, you'll experience a boost in energy and relief from digestive discomfort. Digestive enzymes promote optimal health by heightening the absorption of vitamins, minerals, and other nutrients from food.

12 Life Ionizer Water Machine
What is the closest you can get to natural and pure water?
The Life Ionizer Water Machine not only Alkalizes your water . . . .
They also Test your water for contaminants and then they match special filters to take out those contaminants!

13 Clean Keto vs Dirty Keto book
Find out the difference between clean and dirty keto.
Available on amazon.

14 Thorne Home Blood/Saliva Testing
Weight Management Test
Symptoms attributed to the need for better weight management include:

- Easy weight gain or difficulty losing weight
- Decreases in lean muscle mass
- Increases in abdominal fat
- Fatigue
- Food or sugar cravings
- Poor tolerance for exercise
- Difficulty sleeping or anxiety in the evening (which can contribute to weight gain)

Gut Health Test
Gut health is a foundation for wellness. Thorne's gut microbiome test gives you a detailed analysis and a personalized plan that targets your GI discomfort and optimizes wellness. The test combines cutting-edge sequencing with Onegevity's Health Intelligence to make meaningful changes.

15 **Weight Loss Water**
You know what to eat. But do you know what to drink?
This is a delicious and tasty high fat low carb drink.
That keeps your Insulin Spike below 15%.

16 Meal Replacement Shakes - Chocolate or Vanilla
Delicious high fat low carb meal replacement shakes
When you don't have time to get a meal.

17 Craving and Impulse Control Capsules
Even felt like sneaking around and devouring your favorite high carb
Snack? Knowing you are not supposed to have it. While fear no more
This all natural craving buster will stop those bad cravings instantly.

18 Best Chemical Detoxer - Xeneplex
Approximately 1 billion pounds of pesticides, herbicides and fungicides are applied each year in the United States, with usage doubling every 10 years. Less than 1% of these toxins applied ever find their way to the target pest. The rest goes into our food, water, air and

soil. Pesticides are carcinogens, mutagens and neurotoxins and can damage the immune system and the endocrine system. Glutathione may support the body in dealing with pesticides.

19 Best Heavy Metal Detoxer - Medicardium

Every day your heart pumps 1,900 gallons of blood through the 100,000 miles of living pipes that make up your circulatory system. Over the course of your life, your heart will pump some 2 billion times moving 48 million gallons of blood through your arteries, capillaries and veins. Unfortunately, heart attacks are the leading cause of death in America. Toxins, infections, stress, poor diet and the effects of aging cause the arteries to become brittle and filled with plaque, and blood to thicken and become harder to move. If you are suffering from circulatory disturbances or simply want to increase and maintain your vitality, then ask your doctor if chelation is right for you. *Data regarding heavy metals taken from: Toxicology of Metals. Edited by Louis Chang, 1996.*

20 Prostate Support - Endosterol

Endosterol suppositories offer state of the art prostate support. Endosterol contains beta-sitosterol, saw palmetto, pumpkin seed, dandelion, ellagic acid and Mg Di-K EDTA. Beta sitosterol is both an aromatase and 5-alpha reductase inhibitor thus decreasing the conversion of testosterone to both estrogen and Di-hydro testosterone. Ellagic acid may support apoptosis in prostates with pathological changes. Due to the rectum's immediate proximity to the prostate, Endosterol may deliver its benefits much more efficiently than oral preparations.

21 5 Steps to Heal Yourself and the Planet

22 Collagen

The Cellulite Cleanse stimulates the circulatory and lymphatic systems to help detoxify your tissues. It helps remove waste materials from connective tissues, preventing water retention and promoting the elimination of unwanted substances!

23 Ketone Meter + Ketone strips - All in One Keto Testing Kit

Whether you are newly diagnosed, embracing the ketogenic lifestyle or have been testing for years you can use this kit to better manage your diabetes and ketone levels

24 Intestinal Cleanser
This product helps to break down waste buildup in the colon and ensure that it is successfully eliminated. This maximizes and preserves the benefits of detoxification! It provides a mild laxative effect, improves the function of the stomach and liver, increases the absorption of vital nutrients, and decreases the absorption of toxins. In doing so, it also *naturally relieves gas*

25 Multivitamin/Multimineral
The world's best Multivitamin/Multimineral because it provides a perfect combination of nutrients to promote optimal health, healing, and weight loss. Two capsules of this delicious powder every day provide 100% RDA of all essential vitamins and minerals. The only way to maintain a well-functioning body is to get 100% nutrition in your daily die

26 Probiotic Blend
Gut health is essential to weight loss and healing! Taking a high-quality probiotic can reduce anxiety, improve mood, control acne, improve immune function, and promote healthy cell renewal. It is also extremely effective against Candida. 10 billion friendly bacteria per serving.

27 Earth Grounding Strap
PERFORMANCE BOOSTING ELECTRICAL GROUNDING: Rubber soles in your sneakers block the flow of electricity from your body to the ground but with Erthe you eliminate electric tension to simulate the benefits of exercising barefoot which may speed up recovery and boost performance.

28 Natural Sleep Aid
This incredible supplement is designed to promote healthy sleep, aid in stress management, and soothe an anxious mind. To achieve these outstanding results, this supplement uses a special blend of all-natural ingredients that encourage deep and restorative sleep. In this supplement, phenibut and 5-HTP are used to support the body's natural production of important sleep hormones and ensure a healthy sleep-wake cycle. Melatonin is used to promote restful sleep while reducing disturbances throughout the night. Together, these powerful ingredients ensure that you get the rest you need.

29 Thyroid / Adrenal support

This powerfully healing product contains a blend of 10 synergistic herbs that work together to support your body's natural production of thyroid hormones. It includes iodine-rich seaweeds like kelp and bladderwrack, stress-relieving herbs like sage and hops, and anti-inflammatory herbs like ashwagandha! This supplement can help you overcome thyroid-related symptoms of weight gain, low energy, fatigue, or depression.

30 Vitamin D

Get the benefits of a day in the sun with one simple supplement! Vitamin D will boost your mood, increase your energy, and improve your full body health. Vitamin D offers many health benefits, including bone strengthening, reduced risk of disease, and immune boosting. It comes in an easily absorbable liquid gel-cap form.

31 Post Work-Out Recovery Shake

The Sport Post-Workout Recovery Shake is designed to replenish the nutrients your body uses while exercising. The Post-Workout Recovery Shake doesn't have healthy fats and fibers that slow down the entry of nutrients into your system. Instead, it has added support for your cells to renew their glycogen stores and repair the damaged caused during a workout. This shake is available in chocolate and vanilla.

32 Essential Greens Delicious

Leafy greens are nature's multivitamin. They're packed with vitamins, minerals, and antioxidants that nourish your body and rejuvenate your mind. We've packed a potent blend of greens like spinach, kale, kombu seaweed, and spirulina into this product. Each time you drink your greens, you'll know your body is getting 100% nutrition.

"If you do something right enough, long enough, the end results are predictable." - Dr. Rick Franks

1. But if I eat fat will I get fat?

Negative because your body will be in fat burning mode Ketosis) . . not fat storing mode (glycolysis). You will be using fat (ketones) to think, walk, talk and move with! And when you use fat . . You lose fat . . .nice. . .and easy.

2. What about the keto flu?
You can avoid the bad effects by drinking Rapid Ketosis and taking Celtic sea salt.

3. I still can't get into ketosis?
a) Tighten up your eating window. OMAD. eat only 1X a day

b) Insomnia will stop you from getting into ketosis. Increase your vagal tone (parasympathetic) by belly breathing. Delta binaural beats.

c) Eat more healthy plant based fats

d) Do a brain reset.

e) Check your thyroid with a free T3 and reverse T3 blood test.

f) Check your adrenals with a functional cortisol blood test. And an adrenal stretch test.

g) Do a colonic. You may have an impaction.

4. How can my weight loss be permanent?
By stopping all die-its and get a live-it program it's called creating an affinity to a way of living . . aka. . . LifeStyle .Commit to a long plan (3 months of mote) in order to discover foods and drinks and exercises and fasting methods that you feel good about. Because that's the only way your weight loss will be permanent and sustainable.

5. Fasting sounds like starving and I don't want to starve!
Fasting is controlled and voluntary . . . Starvation is not controlled or voluntary . . .so no worries.

6. Will I have saggy skin if I lose a lot of weight?
Negative . . . not if you lose it with InsulThin Keto/fasting . . Because if you remember the Holocaust and POWs they had no sagging skin because their bodies utilized the excess skin as fuel. Of course that was uncontrolled fasting . . yours will be controlled with the same outcome.

7. But I will have "overwhelming hunger!"
Negative - because God built in to us counter regulatory hormones. Like leptin (the I am full hormone) which goes up during fasting and ghrelin (the I am hungry hormone) which goes down during fasting.

Also adrenalin goes up for energy and growth hormone and BDNF and cortisol for clarity and focus of our minds when we are in a fasted state.

8. Will I become "anorexic"?
Negative - Anorexia is an aberrant psychological disease. We will assume you have all your cognitive abilities and consequently will not be privy to that psychological disorder.

9. But I heard my brain needs 130 grams of carbs a day?
NEGATIVE - If you were in glycolysis (sugar burner) than yes you would need that many carbs. . . .But we are in ketosis and burn fat and use ketones primarily in our brains.

10. Does coffee break a fast?
Black coffee provides a myriad of health benefits, from enhancing fatty acid mobilization from adipose tissue and enhancing cognitive alertness to enhancing metabolism. If you're using a French press, and not a paper filter, a lot of the cholesterols in the coffee can get transported into the blood-brain barrier more easily. And so, coffee— without butter, coconut oil, or any superfood creamers— will actually assist a fast, not harm it.

There are some researchers like Dr. Satchin Panda who hypothesize that the taste of anything, including coffee, can cause this release of incretin hormones or other digestive hormones from the digestive tract that may either make you hungry or may disrupt some of the circadian rhythm benefits of fasting, or may decrease even potentially some of the autophagy benefits of fasting, but I've never seen research that shows that to be the case. And I think that in most cases, coffee, tea, sparkling water, or even non-calorie sources of sweeteners like stevia, for example, in water or in your beverages, is just fine and does not hurt or harm your fast.

Long story short: if it has calories in it, it breaks your fast, and if not, it doesn't. That simple.

11. Is MCT oil better than Coconut Oil?
Negative. MCT oil is missing lauric acid and that is the most studied and most impactful for ketosis. You want coconut oil because it has all the MCT's.

12. How can I get better sleep while fasting?

It's an all too familiar feeling. It's the first night of your fast and there you are, lying awake, chewing on the inside your cheeks thinking about food. Sometimes it's because you're carbohydrate deprived, your serotonin and melatonin are low, your nervous system is stuck in fight-or-flight mode, and sometimes it's because you're just plain hungry. But more often than not it's simply because your body can get by on less sleep while fasting. Use Solutions 4 sleep capsules - available by calling 706.594.9186

13. Can I still train while fasting?

Absolutely Yes you can train and you will probably have more intense workouts because of the counter regulatory hormones: adrenaline Growth hormone and testosterone!

14. Are there any ways of enhancing the benefits of fasting?

Yes. Get a bag of Rapid Ketosis and it will drive you deeper and that will enhance autophagy and apoptosis- cleaning and upregulating your cells.

15. Is a low carb diet the same thing as fasting?

Absolutely not! Low carb will lower your BMI. that's the rate at which you use food energy. And you become a BMI turtle, your metabolic rate will be so slow - you could just look at a pizza and gain weight!

16. Can I Drink Alcohol on the InsulThin Diet?

Yes. "Even though there are [often] carbs in alcohol, you can still drink it in limited amounts," Drinks that are low in sugar and carbs are as follows:

Here's what each alcoholic drink contains, carb-wise:

Dry Wines = Insulin Friendly Wines

Tequila: has 0 carbs and 0 sugar in one shot

Spirits: gin, rum, vodka, whiskey, 1.5 fluid ounce (fl oz), 0 g carbs (1 serving)

Red dry wine, 5 fl oz, 4 g carbs (1 serving)

White wine, 5 fl oz, 4 g carbs (1 serving)

Light beer, 12 fl oz, 6 g carbs (Stick to half of a beer if this is your choice.)

17. Will the InsulThin Diet Give Me Kidney Stones?

The development of kidney stones is certainly a concern if you're going to stay dirty keto in which you're eating more protein. So you should do the 4-1-1 Plan as soon as you reach your goals. You also need to stay hydrated and replenish electrolytes (with celtic sea salt). "If not, this can increase your risk of side effects like stones,

18. How Might the InsulThin Diet Affect My Period?
There's a possibility you may see a change in menstruation. "Studies on younger women who eat keto for an extended period of time end up with irregular periods or missed periods, reason being periods are a route of elimination, and when you break down fats, you open up more toxic load. Because fats hold toxins. And the increased toxic load could upset your periods. On the other side of the spectrum, there is limited evidence that for women with polycystic ovary syndrome (PCOS), a ketogenic diet may improve their hormonal balance. The small study, published in *Nutrition & Metabolism*, found that a small group of women with PCOS who followed a keto diet for 24 weeks lost 12 percent of their body weight and reduced testosterone and insulin levels.

19. How Will the InsulThin Diet Affect Your Cholesterol Levels?
You have to understand that cholesterols are lipoproteins and their job is to help escort acidic toxins out of your body. They cocoon acid wastes so they wont hurt you, and guide them safely to your liver. So that said do not be concerned with cholesterol numbers, because they will normalize once the toxins are out of your body.

20. Can the InsulThin Diet Reverse Type 2 Diabetes?
Virtually in all cases . . Re-read this book.

21. Can I do InsulThin if I do not have a gallbladder?
Yes. You will need to take a special food enzyme with bile in it . .. since you can't store any. It's called Super Enzyme and you can get it here.

REFERENCES -

Evidence based Clinical Studies

"Our reality should not be limited by the perceptions we currently use"
-Paul Stamets

Chapter 1
1. Perlmutter D. Brain Wash: Detox Your Mind for Clearer Thinking, Deeper Relationships and Lasting Happiness. Hachette UK; 2020 Jan 16.
2. Gustafson C. David Perlmutter, MD: The dynamic brain, 1 cite. Integrative Medicine: A Clinician's Journal. 2017 Apr;16(2):22 – 27.
3. Feeney N. Pentagon: 7 in 10 Youths Would Fail to Qualify for Military Service, 9 cites. Time. June. 2014 Jun;29.
4. OVERSPEND I. Bad diets killing more people globally than tobacco, study finds.
5. Raghupathi W, Raghupathi V. An empirical study of chronic diseases in the United States: a visual analytics approach to public health, 61 cites. International journal of environmental research and public health. 2018 Mar;15(3):431. doi: 10.3390/ijerph15030431
6. Calihan, Jennifer. "The economic burden of obesity and diabetes." Web blog post. Diet Doctor. www.dietdoctor.com.
7. CDC. "Obesity and Overweight." Web post. National Center of Health Statistics. cdc.gov.
8. "NCI Dictionary of Cancer Terms." Web post. National Cancer Institute at the National Institute of Health, USA. www.cancer.gov
9. Masood W, Uppaluri KR. Ketogenic Diet, 11 cites. InStatPearls [Internet] 2019 Mar 21. StatPearls Publishing.
10. Felman, Adam. "Does the ketogenic diet work for type 2 diabetes?" Web blog post. Medical News

Today. www.medicalnewstoday.com

11. "Standard American Diet." Web blog post. NutritionFacts.org. nutritionfacts.org.

12. "New theory on how insulin resistance, metabolic disease begin." Web blog post. Science Daily.

13. www.sciencedaily.com

14. "Analysis of new studies including 250,000 people confirms sugar-sweetened drinks are linked to overweight and obesity in children and adults." Web blog post. Science Daily. sciencedaily.com

15. Wilcox G. Insulin and insulin resistance, 1064 cites, USA, 2005. Clinical biochemist reviews, 2005; 26(2):19.

16. CDC. "New CDC report: More than 100 million Americans have diabetes or prediabetes." Web post. National Center of Health Statistics. www.cdc.gov.

17. Tuso P. Prediabetes and lifestyle modification: time to prevent a preventable disease, 111 cites. The Permanente Journal. 2014;18(3):88. doi: 10.7812/TPP/14-002

18. Fung, Jason. "Dr Jason Fung - Understanding And Treating Type 2 Diabetes." YouTube Post. Dr. Jason Fung. Dr Jason Fung YouTube Channel. 20 January. 2019. Web. 20 January. 2019.

19. "Genetic study shows evidence that insulin causes obesity." Web blog post.

20. Diabetes.Co.UK. www.diabetes.co.uk.

21. 19. Sanders FW, Griffin JL. De novo lipogenesis in the liver in health and disease: more than just a shunting yard for glucose, 158 cites. Biological Reviews. 2016 May;91(2):452-68. doi: 10.1111/brv.12178

22. 20. "Nonalcoholic fatty liver disease." Web blog post. Mayo Clinic Staff. www.mayoclinic.org.

23. "Leptin & Insulin Resistance Balancing Tips w/ Jason Fung, MD." YouTube Post. High Intensity Health. High Intensity Health YouTube Channel. 4 April. 2018. Web. 4 April. 2018.

24. Fung, Jason. "Insulin causes insulin resistance." Web blog post. Diet Doctor.

25. www.dietdoctor.com. 3 years ago.

26."The Impact of Non-Alcoholic Fatty Pancreas Disease on Outcome of Acute Pancreatitis." Web post. US National Library of Medicine. www.clinicaltrials.gov. 2 years ago.

27. Eenfeldt, Andreas. Fung, Jason. "The Perfect Treatment for Type 2 Diabetes." YouTube Post. Dr. Jason Fung. Dr Jason Fung YouTube Channel. 17 June. 2015. Web. 17 June. 2015.

28."Gluconeogenesis." Web post. Wikipedia – The free Encyclopedia.

29.www.en.encyclopedia.org.

30.26. "Foie Gras: Cruelty to Ducks and Geese." Web blog post. People for the Ethical Treatment of Animals (PETA). www.peta.org.

31. 27. Marmot M, Steptoe A. Whitehall II and ELSA: Integrating epidemiological and psychobiological approaches to the assessment of biological 335 indicators, 15 cites. InBiosocial surveys 2008. National Academies Press (US).

32. Bilyeu, Tom. "The Shocking Truth About The Keto Diet | Dom D'Agostino on Health Theory." YouTube Post. Tom Bilyeu. Tom Bilyeu YouTube Channel. 25 October. 2018. Web. 25 October. 2018.

33. Berg JM, Tymoczko JL, Stryer L. Glycolysis is an energy-conversion pathway in many organisms, 42 cites. Biochemistry. 5th ed. New York: WH Freeman. 2002.

34."How Much Sugar Do You Eat?" Web post. New Hampshire Department of Health and Human Services. www.dhhs.nh.gov.

35. Webster's New International Dictionary of the English Language, 2nd ed. (1937) Merriam Company, Springfield, Mass.

36.Phinney, Stephen & Team. "Nutritional Ketosis and Ketogenic Diet FAQ" Web blog post.

37. Virta. www.virtahealth.com

38. Hue L, Taegtmeyer H. The Randle cycle revisited: a new head for an old hat, 543 cites. American Journal of Physiology-Endocrinology and Metabolism. 2009 Sep; 297(3):E578- 91. doi:

10.1152/ajpendo.00093.2009

39.Holesh JE, Martin A. Physiology, Carbohydrates. InStatPearls [Internet] 2019 Jun 18. StatPearls Publishing.

40.Dowshen, Steven. "Carbohydrates and Diabetes." Web post. Teens Health for Nemours. www.kidshealth.org

41. Pesta DH, Samuel VT. A high-protein diet for reducing body fat: mechanisms and possible caveats, 136 cites. Nutrition & metabolism. 2014 Dec;11(1):53. doi: 10.1186/1743-7075-11-53

336

42."Glucogenic amino acid" Web post. Wikipedia – The free Encyclopedia.

43.www.en.encyclopedia.org.

44.Dovey, Dana. "High-Protein Diet Reduces Alzheimer's Disease Risk in Older Adults Study Finds". Web blog post. Tech and Science. www.newsweek.com

45.De Widt, Lynda. "Researchers link Alzheimer's gene to Type 3 diabetes". Web blog post.

46.Mayo Clinic. www.newsnetwork.mayoclinic.org.

47.Vagelatos NT, Eslick GD. Type 2 diabetes as a risk factor for Alzheimer's disease: the confounders, interactions, and neuropathology associated with this relationship, 216 cites. Epidemiologic reviews. 2013 Jan 1;35(1):152-60. doi.org/10.1093/epirev/mxs012

48.Mujica-Parodi LR, Amgalan A, Sultan SF, Antal B, Sun X, Skiena S, Lithen A, Adra N, Ratai EM, Weistuch C, Govindarajan ST. Diet modulates brain network stability, a biomarker for brain aging, in young adults. Proceedings of the National Academy of Sciences. 2020 Mar 3. doi.org/10.1073/pnas.1913042117

49.Kawahara M, Kato-Negishi M. Link between aluminum and the pathogenesis of Alzheimer's disease: the integration of the aluminum and amyloid cascade hypotheses,

50.350 cites. International journal of Alzheimer's disease. 2011;2011. doi:

10.4061/2011/276393

51. "NIH study shows how insulin stimulates fat cells to take in glucose". Web post. National Institutes of Health – Turning Discovery into Health. www.nih.gov. 10 years ago.
337

52.44. Freudenrich, Craig. "How Fat Cells Work". Web blog post. How Stuff Works.

53. www.science.howstuffworks.com

54.Neuschwander-Tetri BA. Non-alcoholic fatty liver disease, 141 cites. BMC medicine. 2017 Dec;15(1):45.

55.Majumder S, Philip NA, Takahashi N, Levy MJ, Singh VP, Chari ST. Fatty pancreas: should we be concerned?, 8 cites. Pancreas. 2017 Nov;46(10):1251. doi: 10.1097/MPA.0000000000000941

56.Loomis AK, Kabadi S, Preiss D, Hyde C, Bonato V, St. Louis M, Desai J, Gill JM, Welsh P, Waterworth D, Sattar N. Body mass index and risk of nonalcoholic fatty liver disease: two electronic health record prospective studies, 72 cites. The Journal of Clinical Endocrinology & Metabolism. 2016 Mar 1;101(3):945-52. doi: 10.1210/jc.2015-3444

57. Gilbert VE. Detection of the liver below the costal margin: comparative value of palpation, light percussion, and auscultatory percussion, 15 cites. Southern medical journal. 1994 Feb;87(2):182-6. DOI: 10.1097/00007611-199402000-00006

58.González-Saldivar G, Rodríguez-Gutiérrez R, Ocampo-Candiani J, González-González JG, Gómez-Flores M. Skin manifestations of insulin resistance: from a biochemical stance to a clinical diagnosis and management, 20 cites. Dermatology and therapy. 2017 Mar 1;7(1):37-51. doi: 10.1007/s13555-016-0160-3

59.Hoffman, Kristine. "How Acanthosis Nigricans Can Indicate Insulin Resistance Or Diabetes". Web blog post. Podiatry Today. www.podiatrytoday.com

60.Cruickshank, Heather & Healthline Editorial Team. "Everything You Need to Know About Fatty Liver".
338

Web blog post. Healthline. www.healthline.com. 10 months ago

61. "Insulin, Brown Fat & Ketones: Dr. Bikman's Recent Interview with Mike Mutzel from High Intensity Health". Web blog post. Insulin IQ. www.insuliniq.com. 2 years ago.

62.Erion KA, Corkey BE. Hyperinsulinemia: a cause of obesity?, 49 cites. Current obesity reports. 2017 Jun 1;6(2):178-86. doi: 10.1007/s13679-017-0261-z

63."Lipohypertrophy". Web post. Wikipedia – The free Encyclopedia. www.en.encyclopedia.org.

64."Medical Definition of Metabolism". Web post. MedicineNet. www.medicinenet.com

65."KetoDiet - Take the guesswork out of following a low-carb diet, lose body fat & feel great!". Web Post. Ketodiet. www.ketodietapp.com

66."DO I NEED TO COUNT CALORIES TO LOSE WEIGHT ON KETO?". Web blog post.

67.PaleoLeap. www.paleoleap.com

68.Akesson, A. Eenfeldt, A. "Ten years of ketogenic research with Dr. Dominic D'Agostino". Web post. DietDoctor. www.dietdoctor.com

69.Fung, J. "Controlling the Body's 'Fat Thermometer'". Web blog post. Medium – Lifestyle. www.medium.com

70.Judge TA, Cable DM. When it comes to pay, do the thin win? The effect of weight on pay for men and women, 159 cites. Journal of Applied Psychology. 2011 Jan;96(1):95. doi: 10.1037/a0020860.

Chapter 2

1. Masood W, Uppaluri KR. Ketogenic Diet, 11 cites. InStatPearls [Internet] 2019 Mar 21. StatPearls Publishing. 339

2. Mullens, A. "Ketogenic diet for mental health: Come for the weight loss, stay for the mental health benefits?" Web post. DietDoctor. www.dietdoctor.com

3. Booth, Stephani. "Want a Better Night's Sleep? The Keto Diet Can Help". HealthNews.

www.healthnews.com

4. "How a Ketogenic Diet Really Affects Your Sex Drive". Web blog post. Perfect Keto.

5. www.perfectketo.com

6. Dashti HM, Mathew TC, Hussein T, Asfar SK, Behbahani A, Khoursheed MA, Al-Sayer HM, Bo-Abbas YY, Al-Zaid NS. Long-term effects of a ketogenic diet in obese patients, 99 cites. Experimental & Clinical Cardiology. 2004;9(3):200.

7. "Fighting Cancer Nutritional Ketosis and Intermittent Fasting". Web blog post. Dominic D'Agostino. www. dominicdagostino.wordpress.com.

8. "The Ketogenic Diet & Alzheimer's and the Brain with Dom D'agostino". YouTube Post. Evolving Past Alzheimer's. Evolving Past Alzheimer's YouTube channel. 12 February. 2018. Web. 12 February. 2018.

9. Shaafi S, Mahmoudi J, Pashapour A, Farhoudi M, Sadigh-Eteghad S, Akbari H. Ketogenic diet provides neuroprotective effects against ischemic stroke neuronal damages, 19 cites. Advanced pharmaceutical bulletin. 2014 Dec;4(Suppl 2):479. doi: 10.5681/apb.2014.071

10. Gunnars, K. "10 Health Benefits of Low-Carb and Ketogenic Diets". Web blog post.

11. Healthline. www.healthline.com

12. "The Science Between the Sheets: Can a Keto Diet Increase Sex Drive?". Web blog post.

340

13. Ketologic. www.ketologic.com

14. Booth, Stephani. "Want a Better Night's Sleep? The Keto Diet Can Help". HealthNews. www.healthnews.com

15. Bostock E, Kirkby KC, Taylor BV. The current status of the ketogenic diet in psychiatry, 19 cites. Frontiers in psychiatry. 2017 Mar 20;8:43. doi: 10.3389/fpsyt.2017.00043

16. Jhonson, Stephen. "Can the keto diet help treat depression? Here's what the science says so far". Big Think. www.bigthink.com

17. Akesson, A. Eenfeldt, A. "Ten years of ketogenic

research with Dr. Dominic D'Agostino". Web post.
DietDoctor. www.dietdoctor.com
18. Yancy WS, Foy M, Chalecki AM, Vernon MC,
Westman EC. A low-carbohydrate, ketogenic diet to
treat type 2 diabetes, 276 cites. Nutrition &
metabolism. 2005 Dec 1;2(1):34. doi: 10.1186/1743-
7075-2-34
19. Dashti HM, Mathew TC, Hussein T, Asfar SK,
Behbahani A, Khoursheed MA, Al-Sayer HM, Bo-
Abbas YY, Al-Zaid NS. Long-term effects of a
ketogenic diet in obese patients, 99 cites.
Experimental & Clinical Cardiology. 2004;9(3):200.
20.Bolla AM, Caretto A, Laurenzi A, Scavini M, Piemonti
L. Low-carb and ketogenic diets in type 1 and type 2
diabetes, 10 cites. Nutrients. 2019 May;11(5):962. doi:
10.3390/nu11050962
21. Paoli A, Rubini A, Volek JS, Grimaldi KA. Beyond

weight loss: a review of the therapeutic uses of very-
low-carbohydrate (ketogenic) diets, 531 cites.
European journal of clinical nutrition. 2013
Aug;67(8):789-96. doi: 10.1038/ejcn.2013.116
341
22. Ruskin. Nathaniel, D. "The Effects of Ketogenic Diets
on Inflammation and Chronic Pain". Web post.
Grantome – NIH. www.grantome.com
23. Fung J. The diabetes code: prevent and reverse type
2 diabetes naturally, 10 cites. Greystone Books Ltd;
2018 Apr 3.
24."Type 1 diabetes". Web blog post. Mayo Clinic Staff.
www.mayoclinic.org.
25. Hellerstein MK. De novo lipogenesis in humans:
metabolic and regulatory aspects, 256 cites.
European journal of clinical nutrition. 1999
Apr;53(1):s53-65. DOI: 10.1038/sj.ejcn.1600744
26.Dharmalingam M, Yamasandhi PG. Nonalcoholic
fatty liver disease and type 2 diabetes mellitus, 10
cites. Indian journal of endocrinology and
metabolism. 2018 May;22(3):421. doi:
10.4103/ijem.IJEM_585_17
27. "Jason Fung New Video Fasting/Obesity/Low Carb".

YouTube Post. Weight Loss Motivation. Weight Loss
Motivation YouTube Channel. 14 January. 2020. Web.
14 January. 2020.

28."Dr. Paul Mason - 'Evidence based keto: How to lose
weight and reverse diabetes'". YouTube Post. Low
Carb Down Under. Low Carb Down Under YouTube
Channel. 14 December. 2019. Web. 14 December.
2019.

29.Hardick, B.J. "The Deadly Connection between
Sugar, Acidity and Inflammation". Web blog post.
DrHardick.com. www.hardick.com. 2 years ago.

30.Boyd, Kierstan. Vemulakonda, G. Atma. "What Is
Diabetic Retinopathy?". Web blog post.

31. American Academy of Ophthalmology.
www.aao.org.com
342

32. Weatherspoon, Deborah. "What's to know about
hemorrhagic stroke?". Web blog post.

33. Medical News Today. www.medicalnewstoday.com

34."Inflammation halts fat-burning". Web blog post.
Science Daily. www.sciencedaily.com

35. "Fight Inflammation to Help Prevent Heart
Disease". Web blog post. Jhons Hopkins Medicine.
www.hopkinsmedicine.org

36."High cholesterol strongly linked to risk of stroke".
Web blog post. Nuffield Department of Population
Health. www.ndph.ox.ac.uk

37. "What Is a TIA?". Web blog post. WebMD.
www.webmd.com

38. Sada K, Nishikawa T, Kukidome D, Yoshinaga T,
Kajihara N, Sonoda K, Senokuchi T, Motoshima H,
Matsumura T, Araki E. Hyperglycemia induces
cellular hypoxia through production of
mitochondrial ROS followed by suppression of
aquaporin-1, 27 cites. PLoS One. 2016;11(7). doi:
10.1371/journal.pone.0158619

39."The importance of voltage and its relationship to
oxygen uptake in the body to maintain good health".
Web blog post. Biohealth Energy Systems Ltd.
www.tennantbiomodulator.ca

40.Schmidt, Darren. James, A. "Lactic Acidosis". Web

blog post. Learn True Health.
41. www.learntruehealth.com
42.35. "75 Different Names For Sugar". Web blog post. CHEAT DAY. www. cheatdaydesign.com
43.Tan, V. "How Sugar Causes Cavities and Destroys Your Teeth". Web blog post.
44.HealthLine. www.healthline.com

343
45."Body Fluids and Fluid Compartments". Web blog post. OER Services – Anatomy and Physiology II. www. courses.lumenlearning.com
46."Limb Loss Statistics". Web blog post. Amputee Coalition. www.amputee-coalition.org
47."WHAT IS THE LEADING CAUSE OF BLINDNESS IN THE UNITED STATES?". Web blog post. Aloha Laser Vision. www.alohalaservision.com
48."Heart Disease and Diabetes". Web blog post. WebMD. www.webmd.com
49."Kidney Failure (ESRD) Causes, Symptoms, & Treatments". Web blog post. American Kidney Fund. www.kidneyfund.org
50.Tun NN, Arunagirinathan G, Munshi SK, Pappachan JM. Diabetes mellitus and stroke: a clinical update, 39 cites. World journal of diabetes. 2017 Jun 15;8(6):235. doi: 10.4239/wjd.v8.i6.235
51. Giovannucci E, Harlan DM, Archer MC, Bergenstal RM, Gapstur SM, Habel LA, Pollak M, Regensteiner JG, Yee D. Diabetes and cancer: a consensus report, 2165 cites. CA: a cancer journal for clinicians. 2010 Jul;60(4):207-21. doi: 10.2337/dc10-0666
52.Tessier FJ. The Maillard reaction in the human body. The main discoveries and factors that affect glycation, 177 cites. Pathologie Biologie. 2010 Jun 1;58(3):214-9. DOI: 10.1016/j.patbio.2009.09.014
53. "10 facts on diabetes". Web blog post. World Health Organization. www.who.int
54.Mandal, Ananya. "History of Diabetes". Web blog post. News Medical Life Sciences.
55. www.news-medical.net
56."Sugar rots you Inside out - Dr Jason Fung".

YouTube Post. My 90lbs weight loss journey. My
344

90lbs weight loss journey YouTube Channel. 30
December. 201.8 Web. 30 December. 2018.
57. "What Is Diabetes?". Web blog post. VisionAware.
www.visionaware.org
58."How Weight Loss Surgery Helps Type 2 Diabetes".
Web blog post. WebMD. www.webmd.com
59.Singh AK, Singh R, Kota SK. Bariatric surgery and
diabetes remission: Who would have thought it?, 20
cites. Indian journal of endocrinology and
metabolism. 2015 Sep;19(5):563. doi: 10.4103/2230-
8210.163113
60.Keidar A. Bariatric surgery for type 2 diabetes
reversal: the risks, 39 cites. Diabetes Care. 2011 May
1;34(Supplement 2):S361-266. doi.org/10.2337/dc11-
s254
61. Shah A, Laferrère B. Diabetes after bariatric surgery,
7 cites. Canadian journal of diabetes. 2017 Aug
1;41(4):401-6. doi: 10.1016/j.jcjd.2016.12.009
62.Thorell A, Hagström-Toft E. Treatment of diabetes
prior to and after bariatric surgery, 19 cites. Journal
of diabetes science and technology. 2012
Sep;6(5):1226-32. doi: 10.1177/193229681200600528
63.Prasad, Vinay. "The 'cancer growing in cancer
medicine': pharma money paid to doctors". Web
blog post. STAT. www.statnews.com
64."Dr. Jason Fung - 'A New Paradigm of Insulin
Resistance'". YouTube Post. Low Carb Down Under.
Low Carb Down Under YouTube Channel. 26 May.
2017. Web. 26 May. 2017.
65."Carbohydrates: How carbs fit into a healthy diet".
Web blog post. Mayo Clinic Staff.
66.www.mayoclinic.org.
67."How Type 2 Diabetes Can Damage Your Body". Web
blog post. Health. www.health.com
345

68.Karlsson T, Rask-Andersen M, Pan G, Höglund J,
Wadelius C, Ek WE, Johansson Å. Contribution of

genetics to visceral adiposity and its relation to cardiovascular and metabolic disease, 6 cites. Nature medicine. 2019 Sep;25(9):1390-5.

69.Veech RL. Ketone esters increase brown fat in mice and overcome insulin resistance in other tissues in the rat, 12 cites. Annals of the New York academy of sciences. 2013 Oct;1302(1). doi: 10.1111/nyas.12222

70.Bennet, Madeline. "The Standard American Diet Will Kill Hundreds of Thousands in 2019. Does Anyone Care?". Web blog post. Balanced. www.balanced.org

71. "Is the Standard American Diet Making You Sad, Sick, and Tired?". Web blog post. The Active Times. www.theactivetimes.com

72. Lenoir M, Serre F, Cantin L, Ahmed SH. Intense sweetness surpasses cocaine reward, 560 cites. PloS one. 2007;2(8). doi: 10.1371/journal.pone.0000698

73. Sullum, Jacob. "Research Shows Cocaine And Heroin Are Less Addictive Than Oreos". Blog post. Forbes. www.forbes.com

74.Didymus J. "Study: High-fructose corn syrup is as addictive as cocaine". Web blog post.

75. Digital Journal. www.digitaljournal.com

76."IS SUGAR ADDICTIVE?". Web blog post. Well Balance. www.wellbalance.ca

77. "Quotes from "Alcoholics Anonymous". Web post. Minnesota Recovery Page. www.minnesotarecovery.info

78.Alcaro A, Huber R, Panksepp J. Behavioral functions of the mesolimbic dopaminergic system: an affective neuroethological perspective, 423 cites. Brain research reviews. 2007 Dec 1;56(2):283-321. doi: 10.1016/j.brainresrev.2007.07.014

346

79.Centers for Disease Control and Prevention. New CDC report: More than 100 million Americans have diabetes or prediabetes, 33 cites. Retrieved from Centers for Disease Control and Prevention: https://www. cdc. gov/media/releases/2017/p0718-diabetesreport. html. 2017 Jul 18.

80.Mammoser, Gigen. "Keto Diet Can Help You Live Longer, Researchers Say". Web blog post.

HealthLine. www.healthline.com

81. Mawer, Rudy. "10 Signs and Symptoms That You're in Ketosis". Web blog post.

82.HealthLine. www.healthline.com

83.Frida, H. K. Eenfeldt, A. "How a keto diet could help you live longer". Web blog post. Diet Doctor. www.dietdoctor.com.

84.Hill, Ansley. "14 Healthy Fats for the Keto Diet (Plus Some to Limit)". Web blog post.

85.HealthLine. www.healthline.com

86.Eriksson KF, Lindgärde F. Prevention of Type 2 (non-insulin-dependent) diabetes mellitus by diet and physical exercise The 6-year Malmö feasibility study, 1581 cites. Diabetologia. 1991 Dec 1;34(12):891-8. DOI: 10.1007/bf00400196

87."Leading Scientists Agree: Current Limits on Saturated Fats No Longer Justified". Web blog post. Nutrition Coalition. www.nutritioncoalition.us

88.Saksuriyongse, T. "Heart Disease and Cancer: The Top 2 Killers in the U.S." Web blog post. AIR – A Verisk Business. www.air-worldwide.com

89."Five Things Monsanto Doesn't Want You to Know About GMOs". Web blog post. Food and Water Watch. www.foodandwaterwatch.org

347

90."U.S. and Monsanto Dominate Global Market for GM Seeds". Web blog post. Organic Consumer Association. www.organicconsumers.org

91. Gillam, C. "How Monsanto manipulates journalists and academics". Web blog post. Support the Guardian. www.theguardian.com

92.Olney JW, Farber NB, Spitznagel E, Robins LN. Increasing brain tumor rates: is there a link to aspartame?, 217 cites. Journal of Neuropathology & Experimental Neurology. 1996 Nov 1;55(11):1115-23. DOI: 10.1097/00005072-199611000-00002

93.King, J. "Effects of Aspartame on the Heart". Web blog post. LIVINGSTRONG.com

94.www.livestrong.com

95."THE REAL TRUTH ABOUT ARTIFICIAL SWEETENERS". Web blog post. MI Smiles Dental.

www.mismilesdental.com

96.Bedwell, S-J. Winderi, A.M. "19 Healthy, High-Fat Foods to Keep You Full and Satisfied". Web blog post. Self. www.self.com

97.Chang CY, Ke DS, Chen JY. Essential fatty acids and human brain, 170 cites. Acta Neurol Taiwan. 2009 Dec 1;18(4):231-41.

98.Zhang J, Liu Q. Cholesterol metabolism and homeostasis in the brain, 198 cites. Protein & cell. 2015 Apr 1;6(4):254-64. doi: 10.1007/s13238-014-0131-3

99.Carter, A. "Lipids, Steroids, and Cholesterol: How They're Connected". Web blog post.

100. Healthline. www.healthline.com

101. JASTRZEBSkI Z, Kortas J, Kaczor K, Antosiewicz J. Vitamin D supplementation causes a decrease in blood cholesterol in professional rowers, 6 cites. Journal of nutritional science and

348

vitaminology. 2016;62(2):88-92. doi: 10.3177/jnsv.62.88.

102. Alberts B, Johnson A, Lewis J, Raff M, Roberts K, Walter P. The lipid bilayer, 47 cites. InMolecular Biology of the Cell. 4th edition 2002. Garland Science.

103. Yeager, S. "13 Healthy High-Fat Foods You Should Eat More". Web blog post. Health. www.health.com

104. Clark, C. Shafipour, P. "Ketogenic Diet Food List: Everything You Need to Know". Web blog post. Ruled.Me. www.ruled.me

105. Calihan, J. Eedfeldt, A. "Ketogenic diet food list – what to buy". Web blog post.

106. DietDoctor. www.dietdoctor.com

107. "Keto vs Fat Adapted - Dr. Mike Grego. DC". YouTube Post. Dr. grego Keto Doc. Dr. grego Keto Doc YouTube Channel. 18 September. 2017. Web. 18 September. 2017.

108. Buppajarntham, S. Junpaparp, P. Salameh, R. Anastasopoulou, C. Staros, E B. Lin, J. "Insulin". Web post. MedScape. www.emedicine.medscape.com

109. Prince A, Zhang Y, Croniger C, Puchowicz M. Oxidative metabolism: glucose versus ketones, 15 cites. InOxygen Transport to Tissue XXXV 2013 (pp. 323-328). Springer, New York, NY. doi: 10.1007/978-1-4614-7411-1_43.

110. Prasad K, Dhar I. Oxidative stress as a mechanism of added sugar-induced cardiovascular disease, 55 cites. International Journal of Angiology. 2014 Dec;23(04):217-26. doi: 10.1055/s-0034-1387169

111.Bookshelf ID. NBK21190. Chapter 21Glycogen Metabolism.

349

112. "Fats and Cholesterol". Web blog post. Harvard T.H Chan – The Nutrition Source. www.hsph.harvard.edu

113. Iqbal MP. Trans fatty acids–A risk factor for cardiovascular disease, 27 cites. Pakistan journal of medical sciences. 2014 Jan;30(1):194. doi: 10.12669/pjms.301.4525

114. DiNicolantonio JJ, O'Keefe JH. Omega-6 vegetable oils as a driver of coronary heart disease: the oxidized linoleic acid hypothesis,13 cites. Open heart. 2018 Oct 1;5(2):e000898. doi.org/10.1136/openhrt-2018-000898

115. Malhotra A, DiNicolantonio JJ, Capewell S. It is time to stop counting calories, and time instead to promote dietary changes that substantially and rapidly reduce cardiovascular morbidity and mortality, 2 cites. doi.org/10.1136/openhrt-2015-000273

116. Food and Drug Administration. A food labeling guide, 36 cites.

117. Higdon J. Essential fatty acids, 18 cites. Linus Pauling Institute-Oregon State University. 2003.

118. "Amino acids". Web post. MedlinePLUS. www. medlineplus.gov

119. Berg JM, Tymoczko JL, Stryer L. Section 16.3. Glucose can be-synthesized from noncarbohydrate precursors, 9 cites. Biochemistry. 2002:479-85.

120. Bender DA. Tricarboxylic acid cycle, 5 cites.

121. "Connections between cellular respiration and other pathways". Web lecture post. Khan Academy. www.khanacademy.org

122. Munawar A, Ali SA, Akrem A, Betzel C. Snake venom peptides: Tools of biodiscovery, 11 cites.
350
Toxins. 2018 Nov;10(11):474. doi: 10.3390/toxins10110474

123. Vick, A. "SNAKE AND SPIDER VENOM ALSO HELP SAVE LIVES". Web blog post. Eureka. www. eureka.criver.com

124. Li Q, Xu M, Cui Y, Huang C, Sun M. Arginine-rich membrane-permeable peptides are seriously toxic, 6 cites. Pharmacology research & perspectives. 2017 Oct 1;5(5). doi: 10.1002/prp2.334

125. Munawar A, Ali SA, Akrem A, Betzel C. Snake venom peptides: Tools of biodiscovery, 11 cites. Toxins. 2018 Nov;10(11):474. doi.org/10.3390/toxins10110474

126. Davis, C. "Busting the Myth of Incomplete Plant-Based Proteins". Web post.

127. Medium. www.medium.com

128. "FUN FACES OF WISCONSIN AGRICULTURE - BEEF ANIMAL'S DIET". PDF web upload. Wisag Classroom. www.wisagclassroom.org

129. "The Game Changers | Official Trailer." YouTube post. The Game Changers. The Game Changers YouTube Channel. 28 June. 2018. Web. 28 June. 2018.

Chapter 3

1. Fung, J. "The common currency in our bodies is not calories – guess what it is?". Web blog post. Diet Doctor. www.dietdoctor.com

2. Teta, Jade. "Want to Lose Fat? Count Your Hormones, Not Your Calories (Part 3)". Web blog post. HuffPost. www.huffpost.com

3. Schwarz NA, Rigby BR, La Bounty P, Shelmadine B, Bowden RG. A review of weight control strategies and their effects on the regulation of hormonal
351

balance, 59 cites. Journal of nutrition and
metabolism. 2011 Jul 28;2011. doi:
10.1155/2011/237932

4. "Why hormones matter more than calories for fat
loss: the role of insulin". Web blog post. Poliquin
Group. www.main.poliquingroup.com

5. Fung, J. "The Biggest Loser FAIL and that ketogenic
study success". Web blog post.

6. Diet Doctor. www.dietdoctor.com

7. Fung, J. "Cutting calories won't solve your weight
issues – do this instead". Web blog post. Diet Doctor.
www.dietdoctor.com

8. Hyman, M. "Why "Skinny Fat" Can Be Worse than
Obesity". Web blog post. Dr. Hyman.
www.drhyman.com

9. Lustig, R. "Fat Chance: Fructose 2.0 by Dr. Robert
Lustig (Transcript)". Web blog post.

10. The Singju Post. www.singjupost.com

11. "Low-Fat Diet Not a Cure-All". Web blog post.
Harvard T.H Chan – The Nutrition Source.
www.hsph.harvard.edu

12. Benton D, Young HA. Reducing calorie intake may
not help you lose body weight, 28 cites. Perspectives
on Psychological Science. 2017 Jun 28. doi:
10.1177/1745691617690878

13. "Leptin & Insulin Resistance Balancing Tips w/ Jason
Fung, MD". YouTube Post. High Intensity Health.
High Intensity Health YouTube Channel. 4 April.
2018. Web. 4 April. 2018.

14. Sotos JF, Tokar NJ. Growth hormone significantly
increases the adult height of children with idiopathic
short stature: comparison of subgroups and benefit,
31 cites. International journal of pediatric

352

endocrinology. 2014 Dec 1;2014(1):15. doi:
10.1186/1687-9856- 2014-15

15. Finn, C. "The Complicated Relationship Between
Testosterone and Muscle Growth". Web blog post.
VICE Media Group. www.vice.com

16. Dfarhud D, Malmir M, Khanahmadi M. Happiness &
health: the biological factors- systematic review

Article, 49 cites. Iranian journal of public health.
2014 Nov;43(11):1468.

17. Bloch M, Meiboom H, Zaig I, Schreiber S, Abramov
L. The use of dehydroepiandrosterone in the
treatment of hypoactive sexual desire disorder: a
report of gender differences, 23 cites. European
Neuropsychopharmacology. 2013 Aug 1;23(8):910-8.
DOI: 10.1016/j.euroneuro.2012.09.004

18. Carter, A. "What to know about insulin and weight
gain". Web blog post. Medical News Today.
www.medicalnewstoday.com

19. Buscemi N, Vandermeer B, Pandya R, Hooton N,
Tjosvold L, Hartling L, Baker G, Vohra S, Klassen T.
Melatonin for treatment of sleep disorders:
summary. InAHRQ evidence report summaries 2004
Nov, 24 cites. Agency for Healthcare Research and
Quality (US).

20.Cafasso, J. Sukkivan, D. "Adrenaline Rush:
Everything You Should Know". Web blog post.
Healthline. www.healthline.com

21. "Love hormone is released during crises". Web post.
Science Daily. www.sciencedaily.com

22.Stephens MA, Wand G. Stress and the HPA axi: Role
of glucocorticoids in alcohol dependence, 287 cites.
Alcohol research: current reviews. 2012.

23. Shors TJ, Leuner B. Estrogen-mediated effects on
depression and memory formation in females, 164
353
cites. Journal of affective disorders. 2003 Mar
1;74(1):85-96.

24."Biology of leptin, the hunger hormone, revealed".
Web post. Science Daily. www.sciencedaily.com

25.Pradhan G, Samson SL, Sun Y. Ghrelin: much more
than a hunger hormone, 123 cites. Current opinion in
clinical nutrition and metabolic care. 2013
Nov;16(6):619. doi: 10.1097/MCO.0b013e328365b9be

26.Russell-Jones D, Khan R. Insulin-associated weight
gain in diabetes–causes, effects and coping
strategies, 424 cites. Diabetes, Obesity and
Metabolism. 2007 Nov;9(6):799- 812. DOI:
10.1111/j.1463-1326.2006.00686.x

27. Gruzdeva O, Borodkina D, Uchasova E, Dyleva Y, Barbarash O. Leptin resistance: underlying mechanisms and diagnosis, 16 cites. Diabetes, metabolic syndrome and obesity: targets and therapy. 2019;12:191. doi: 10.2147/DMSO.S182406

28.Paintal AS. A study of gastric stretch receptors. Their role in the peripheral mechanism of satiation of hunger and thirst, 315 cites. The Journal of physiology. 1954 Nov 29;126(2):255-70. doi: 10.1113/jphysiol.1954.sp005207

29.Moran TH. Cholecystokinin and satiety: current perspectives, 303 cites. Nutrition. 2000 Oct 1;16(10):858-65. DOI: 10.1016/s0899-9007(00)00419-6

30. Holst JJ. The physiology of glucagon-like peptide 1, 2554 cites. Physiological reviews. 2007 Oct;87(4):1409-39. DOI: 10.1152/physrev.00034.2006

31. Batterham RL, Heffron H, Kapoor S, Chivers JE, Chandarana K, Herzog H, Le Roux CW, Thomas EL, Bell JD, Withers DJ. Critical role for peptide YY in 354
protein-mediated satiation and body-weight regulation, 610 cites. Cell metabolism. 2006 Sep 1;4(3):223- 33. DOI: 10.1016/j.cmet.2006.08.001

32. "Investigating the Role of Ghrelin in Regulating Appetite and Energy Intake in Patients Following Bariatric Surgery (BARI-INSIGHT) (BARI-INSIGHT)". Web post. NIH U.S National Library of Medicine - ClinicalTrials.Gov. www.clinicaltrials.gov

33. Druce MR, Wren AM, Park AJ, Milton JE, Patterson M, Frost G, Ghatei MA, Small C, Bloom SR. Ghrelin increases food intake in obese as well as lean subjects, 411 cites. International journal of obesity. 2005 Sep;29(9):1130-6. DOI: 10.1038/sj.ijo.0803001

34.Klok MD, Jakobsdottir S, Drent ML. The role of leptin and ghrelin in the regulation of food intake and body weight in humans: a review, 1111 cites. Obesity reviews. 2007 Jan;8(1):21-34. DOI: 10.1111/j.1467-789X.2006.00270.x

35. Cummings DE. Ghrelin and the short-and long-term

regulation of appetite and body weight, 673 cites. Physiology & behavior. 2006 Aug 30;89(1):71-84. DOI: 10.1016/j.physbeh.2006.05.022

36.Hansen TK, Dall R, Hosoda H, Kojima M, Kangawa K, Christiansen JS, Jørgensen JO. Weight loss increases circulating levels of ghrelin in human obesity, 627. Clinical endocrinology. 2002 Feb;56(2):203-6. DOI: 10.1046/j.0300-0664.2001.01456.x

37. Müller TD, Nogueiras R, Andermann ML, Andrews ZB, Anker SD, Argente J, Batterham RL, Benoit SC, Bowers CY, Broglio F, Casanueva FF. Ghrelin, 452 cites. Molecular metabolism. 2015 Jun 1;4(6):437-60. DOI: 10.1016/j.molmet.2015.03.005

38."The Best High-fat Foods to Eat on the Keto Diet". Web blog post. MODIUS. www. us.modiushealth.com 355

39.Woolf SH, Schoomaker H. Life expectancy and mortality rates in the United States, 1959-2017, 26 cites. Jama. 2019 Nov 26;322(20):1996-2016. DOI: 10.1001/jama.2019.16932

40.Woolf SH, Chapman DA, Buchanich JM, Bobby KJ, Zimmerman EB, Blackburn SM. Changes in midlife death rates across racial and ethnic groups in the United States: systematic analysis of vital statistics, 46 cites. Bmj. 2018 Aug 15;362:k3096. doi.org/10.1136/bmj.k3096

41. Christensen, J. "US life expectancy is still on the decline. Here's why". Web blog post.

42.CNN Health. www.edition.cnn.com

43."Statistics on Dieting and Eating Disorders". Web PDF upload. MonteNido. www.montenido.com

44.The Columbus Weight Loss Clinic. E - Store. www.thecolumbusweightlossclinic.com

45.Puchalska P, Crawford PA. Multi-dimensional roles of ketone bodies in fuel metabolism, signaling, and therapeutics, 242 cites. Cell metabolism. 2017 Feb 7;25(2):262-84. doi: 10.1016/j.cmet.2016.12.022

46."Ketones: The Furth Macronutrient with Dr. Dominic D'Agostino". Web podcast.

47.FxMedicine. www.fxmedicine.com.au

48.Hasselbalch SG, Knudsen GM, Jakobsen JO, Hageman

LP, Holm S, Paulson OB. Blood-brain barrier permeability of glucose and ketone bodies during short-term starvation in humans, 123 cites. American Journal of Physiology-Endocrinology and Metabolism. 1995 Jun 1;268(6):E1161-6. DOI: 10.1152/ajpendo.1995.268.6.E1161

49."Dr. Benjamin Bikman - 'Insulin vs. Ketones - The Battle for Brown Fat'". YouTube Post. Low Carb

356

Down Under. Low Carb Down Under YouTube Channel. 17 March. 2017. Web. 17 March. 2017.

50."Insulin, Brown Fat & Ketones: Dr. Bikman's Recent Interview with Mike Mutzel from High Intensity Health". Web blog post. INSULIN IQ. www.insuliniq.com

51. "Ketogenic Q&A Part 2: Ketones, Fasting, and the Brain - Dominic D'Agostino, PhD". YouTube Post. Metagenics Institute. Metagenics Institute YouTube Channel. 7 September. 2018. Web. 7 September. 2018

52.Wolpert, S. "Dieting does not work, UCLA researchers report". Web blog post.

53. Newsroom. www.newsroom.ucla.edu

54.Dashti HM, Mathew TC, Hussein T, Asfar SK, Behbahani A, Khoursheed MA, Al-Sayer HM, Bo-Abbas YY, Al-Zaid NS. Long-term effects of a ketogenic diet in obese patients, 99 cites. Experimental & Clinical Cardiology. 2004;9(3):200.

55.Wilen, C J. "The 95%: Why Women embrace diets that don't work". Web PDF upload as

56.Honors Essay. www.globalstudies.unc.edu

Chapter 4

1. O'Hearn, A. "Babies thrive under a ketogenic metabolism". Web blog post. The Ketogenic Diet for Health. www.ketotic.org

2. Gustin, A. "Here's What Research Says About Keto While Breastfeeding". Web blog post. Perfect Keto. www.perfectketo.com

3. Den Daas C, Häfner M, de Wit J. Out of Sight, Out of Mind, 15 cites. Experimental psychology. 2013. doi: 10.1027/1618-3169/a000201

4. "What's in your drinking water?". Web blog post. Water & Health. www.freshlysqueezedwater.org.uk
357

5. AlAzmi A, AlHamdan H, Abualezz R, Bahadig F, Abonofal N, Osman M. Patients' knowledge and attitude toward the disposal of medications, 12 cites. Journal of pharmaceutics. 2017;2017. doi: 10.1155/2017/8516741

6. Tanaka Y, Saihara Y, Izumotani K, Nakamura H. Daily ingestion of alkaline electrolyzed water containing hydrogen influences human health, including gastrointestinal symptoms, 2 cites. Medical gas research. 2018 Oct;8(4):160. doi: 10.4103/2045- 9912.248267

7. Ferriss, T. "Dom D'Agostino on Fasting, Ketosis, and the End of Cancer (#117)". Web blog post. Tim Ferriss. www.tim.blog

8. Clancy PM, Kennedy GT, Lynch JE. Fast and abstinence, 8 cites. New Catholic Encyclopedia. 1967;5:632-35.

9. Williams, J. "Ramadan 2019: 9 questions about the Muslim holy month you were too embarrassed to ask". Web blog post. Vox. www.vox.com

10. Abramson, A. "Here's Why People Fast on Yom Kippur". Web blog post. Time. www.time.com

11. "Fasting on Mahashivratri: Why you should do it". Web blog post. The Art of Living. www.artofliving.org

12. Berbesque JC, Marlowe FW, Shaw P, Thompson P. Hunter–gatherers have less famine than agriculturalists, 48 cites. Biology Letters. 2014 Jan 31;10(1):20130853. doi: 10.1098/rsbl.2013.0853

13. Broadfoot-Duke, M. "Starvation Diet Puts Worm Lifespan on 'Pause'". Web blog post.

14. Futurity. www.futurity.org
358

15. Haridy, Rich. "Harvard study uncovers why fasting can lead to a longer and healthier life". Web blog post. New Atlas. www.newatlas.com

16. Everts, S. "Yoshinori Ohsumi wins 2016 Nobel Prize

in Physiology or Medicine". Web blog post. Chemical & Engineering News. www.cen.acs.org

17. Nakamura S, Yoshimori T. Autophagy and longevity, 48 cites. Molecules and cells. 2018 Jan 31;41(1):65. doi: 10.14348/molcells.2018.2333

18. Yee C, Yang W, Hekimi S. The intrinsic apoptosis pathway mediates the pro-longevity response to mitochondrial ROS in C. elegans, 261 cites. Cell. 2014 May 8;157(4):897- 909. doi: 10.1016/j.cell.2014.02.055

19. Anton S, Leeuwenburgh C. Fasting or caloric restriction for healthy aging, 78 cites. doi: 10.1016/j.exger.2013.04.011

20.Li L, Wang Z, Zuo Z. Chronic intermittent fasting improves cognitive functions and brain structures in mice, 71 cites. PloS one. 2013;8(6). doi: 10.1371/journal.pone.0066069

21. Cheng CW, Adams GB, Perin L, Wei M, Zhou X, Lam BS, Da Sacco S, Mirisola M, Quinn DI, Dorff TB, Kopchick JJ. Prolonged fasting reduces IGF-1/PKA to promote hematopoietic-stem-cell-based regeneration and reverse immunosuppression, 245 cites. Cell stem cell. 2014 Jun 5;14(6):810-23. doi.org/10.1016/j.stem.2014.04.014

22."Fasting helps improve mood, sex and sleep". Web blog post. ETimes. www.timesofindia.indiatimes.com

23. Quattrini S, Pampaloni B, Brandi ML. Natural mineral waters: chemical characteristics and health effects, 35 cites. Clinical cases in mineral and bone

359

metabolism. 2016 Sep;13(3):173. doi: 10.11138/ccmbm/2016.13.3.173

24."Is Celtic Salt Suitable as an Electrolyte Supplement?". Web blog post. Seventh Wave. www.seventhwaveuk.com

25.Witkowski JA. Dr. Carrel's immortal cells, 105 cites. Medical history. 1980 Apr;24(2):129- 42. doi: 10.1017/s0025727300040126

26.Papandreou D, Karavolias C, Arvaniti F, Kafeza E, Sidawi F. Fasting ghrelin levels are decreased in obese subjects and are significantly related with insulin resistance and body mass index, 6 cites. Open access Macedonian journal of medical sciences. 2017 Oct 15;5(6):699. doi: 10.3889/oamjms.2017.182

27. Chan JL, Heist K, DePaoli AM, Veldhuis JD, Mantzoros CS. The role of falling leptin levels in the neuroendocrine and metabolic adaptation to short-term starvation in healthy

28.men, 669 cites. The Journal of clinical investigation. 2003 May 1;111(9):1409-21. doi: 10.1172/JCI200317490

29.27. Maalouf M, Sullivan PG, Davis L, Kim DY, Rho JM. Ketones inhibit mitochondrial production of reactive oxygen species production following glutamate excitotoxicity by increasing NADH oxidation, 305 cites. Neuroscience. 2007 Mar 2;145(1):256-64. doi: 10.1016/j.neuroscience.2006.11.065

29.Berg JM, Tymoczko JL, Stryer L. Triacylglycerols are highly concentrated energy stores, 23 cites. Biochemistry. 2002;5.

30.Chansky M, Haddad G. Acute diabetic emergencies, hypoglycemia, and glycemic control, 1 cite. InCritical Care Medicine 2008 Jan 1 (pp. 1245-1267). Mosby. 360

31. Davis LM, Pauly JR, Readnower RD, Rho JM, Sullivan PG. Fasting is neuroprotective following traumatic brain injury, 134 cites. Journal of neuroscience research. 2008 Jun;86(8):1812-22. doi: 10.1002/jnr.21628.

32. Bakhach M, Shah V, Harwood T, Lappe S, Bhesania N, Mansoor S, Alkhouri N. The protein-sparing modified fast diet: an effective and safe approach to induce rapid weight loss in severely obese adolescents, 10 cites. Global pediatric health. 2016 Jan 22;3 doi: 10.1177/2333794X15623245

33. Wang M, Wang Q, Whim MD. Fasting induces a form of autonomic synaptic plasticity that prevents hypoglycemia, 15 cites. Proceedings of the National Academy of Sciences. 2016 May 24;113(21):E3029-38. doi: 10.1073/pnas.1517275113

34. Higdon JV, Frei B. Tea catechins and polyphenols: health effects, metabolism, and antioxidant functions, 1816 cites. DOI: 10.1080/10408690390826464

35. Boswell-Smith V, Spina D, Page CP. Phosphodiesterase inhibitors, 408 cites. British journal of pharmacology. 2006 Jan;147(S1):S252-7. doi:10.1038/sj.bjp.0706495

36."6 Tips To Differentiate Hunger vs. Thirst". Web blog post. Corporate Wellness Magazine. www.corporatewellnessmagazine.com

37. Moroney, B. "The Dreaded Jarisch-Herxheimer Reaction". Web blog post. AMJ. www.amajordifference.com

38.Brett. MicKay, K. "The Herschel Walker Workout". Web blog post. Fitness, Health & Sports, Sports. www.artofmanliness.com
361

39.Santilli V, Bernetti A, Mangone M, Paoloni M. Clinical definition of sarcopenia, 221 cites. Clinical cases in mineral and bone metabolism. 2014 Sep;11(3):177.

40.Lager I. The insulin-antagonistic effect of the counterregulatory hormones, 65 cites. Journal of internal medicine. Supplement. 1991;735:41-7.

41. Mattson MP. Energy intake, meal frequency, and health: a neurobiological perspective, 266 cites. Annu. Rev. Nutr.. 2005 Jul 11;25:237-60. DOI: 10.1146/annurev.nutr.25.050304.092526

42.Mattson MP. Energy intake, meal frequency, and health: a neurobiological perspective, 266 cites. Annu. Rev. Nutr.. 2005 Jul 11;25:237-60. DOI: 10.1146/annurev.nutr.25.050304.092526

43.Teng CT, Li Y, Stockton P, Foley J. Fasting induces the expression of PGC-1α and ERR isoforms in the outer stripe of the outer medulla (OSOM) of the mouse kidney, 10 cites. PloS one. 2011;6(11). doi: 10.1371/journal.pone.0026961

44.Liang H, Ward WF. PGC-1α: a key regulator of energy metabolism, 859 cites. Advances in physiology education. 2006 Dec;30(4):145-51. DOI:

10.1152/advan.00052.2006

45.Zhu Y, Yan Y, Gius DR, Vassilopoulos A. Metabolic regulation of Sirtuins upon fasting and the implication for cancer, 28 cites. Current opinion in oncology. 2013 Nov;25(6):630. doi: 10.1097/01.cco.0000432527.49984.a3

46.Lee D, Martinez B, Crocker DE, Ortiz RM. Fasting increases the phosphorylation of AMPK and expression of sirtuin1 in muscle of adult male northern elephant seals (Mirounga angustirostris), 5

362

cites. Physiological reports. 2017 Feb;5(4):e13114. DOI: 10.14814/phy2.13114

47.Cabeca, Anna. "Fasting, mTOR, Autophagy... And The Importance Of The Feast!". Web blog post. The Girlfriend Doctor - Dr. Anna Cabeca. www.drannacabeca.com

48."Dr. Peter Attia: Fasting, Autophagy, and mTOR Inhibition – High Intensity Health". Web blog post. PODCAST NOTES. www.podcastnotes.org

49.Sengupta S, Peterson TR, Laplante M, Oh S, Sabatini DM. mTORC1 controls fasting- induced ketogenesis and its modulation by ageing, 429 cites. Nature. 2010 Dec;468(7327):1100-4. doi:10.1038/nature09584

50.Longo VD, Panda S. Fasting, circadian rhythms, and time-restricted feeding in healthy lifespan, 249 cites. Cell metabolism. 2016 Jun 14;23(6):1048-59. doi: 10.1016/j.cmet.2016.06.001

51. ""Mitochondrial DNA variation in Human Origins and Disease". YouTube Post. Case Western Reserve University. Case Western Reserve University YouTube Channel. 20 July. 2016. Web. 20 July. 2016.

52. Stefano GB, Bjenning C, Wang F, Wang N, Kream RM. Mitochondrial Heteroplasmy, 6 cites. InMitochondrial Dynamics in Cardiovascular Medicine 2017 (pp. 577-594). Springer, Cham. doi: 10.1007/978-3-319-55330-6_30.

53. "The story of Angus Barbieri, who went 382 days without eating". Web blog post.

54.Diabetes.co.uk – The Global Diabetes Community. www.diabetes.co.uk

55. Kostraba B, Wu YN, Kao PC, Stark C, Yen SC, Roh J. Muscle activation pattern during self-propelled treadmill walking, 1 cite. Journal of physical therapy

363

science. 2018;30(8):1069-72. doi: 10.1589/jpts.30.1069
56."Major fat-burning discovery". Web blog post. Harvard Health Publishing – Harvard Medical School. www.health.harvard.edu
57. Hensrud, D. "Can I boost my metabolism to lose weight?". Web blog post. Healthy Lifestyle – Weight Loss. www.mayoclinic.org
58."Exercise Reverses Aging In Human Skeletal Muscle". Web blog post. Science Daily. www.sciencedaily.com
59.Husak JF, Irschick DJ. Steroid use and human performance: lessons for integrative biologists, 17 cites. Integrative and comparative biology. 2009 Oct 1;49(4):354-64. doi.org/10.1093/icb/icp015
60.Velloso CP. Regulation of muscle mass by growth hormone and IGF-I, 369 cites. British journal of pharmacology. 2008 Jun 1;154(3):557-68. doi: 10.1038/bjp.2008.153
61. "Wake Up". YouTube Post. DDP Yoga. DDP Yoga YouTube Channel. 20 September. 2011. Web. 20 September. 2011.
62."What is HIIT? 7 Proven HIIT Benefits and How to Do It Properly | The Health Nerd". YouTube Post. The Health Nerd. The Health Nerd YouTube Channel. 1 July. 2017. Web. 1 July. 2017.

Chapter 5
1. Sender R, Fuchs S, Milo R. Revised estimates for the number of human and bacteria cells in the body, 1557 cites. PLoS biology. 2016 Aug 19;14(8):e1002533. doi: 10.1371/journal.pbio.1002533
2. Grice EA, Segre JA. The human microbiome: our second genome, 390 cites. Annual review of

364

genomics and human genetics. 2012 Sep 22;13:151-

70. doi: 10.1146/annurev- genom-090711-163814

3. "What is a gene?". Web post. NIH. U.S National Library of Medicine. www.ghr.nlm.nih.gov

4. Strandwitz P. Neurotransmitter modulation by the gut microbiota, 74 cites. Brain research. 2018 Aug 15;1693:128-33. doi: 10.1016/j.brainres.2018.03.015.

5. Hadhazy, A. "Think Twice: How the Gut's "Second Brain" Influences Mood and Well- Being". Web blog post. Scientific American. www.scientificAmerican.com

6. Vighi G, Marcucci F, Sensi L, Di Cara G, Frati F. Allergy and the gastrointestinal system, 214 cites. Clinical & Experimental Immunology. 2008 Sep;153:3-6. doi: 10.1111/j.1365- 2249.2008.03713.x

7. Underwood, E. "Your gut is directly connected to your brain, by a newly discovered neuron circuit". Web blog post. Science. www.sciencemag.org

8. Kulecka M, Paziewska A, Zeber-Lubecka N, Ambrozkiewicz F, Kopczynski M, Kuklinska U, Pysniak K, Gajewska M, Mikula M, Ostrowski J. Prolonged transfer of feces from the lean mice modulates gut microbiota in obese mice, 39 cites. Nutrition & metabolism. 2016 Dec 1;13(1):57. doi: 10.1186/s12986-016-0116-8

9. Ahima RS. Digging deeper into obesity, 208 cites. The Journal of clinical investigation. 2011 Jun 1;121(6):2076-9. DOI: 10.1172/JCI58719

10. Mu Q, Kirby J, Reilly CM, Luo XM. Leaky gut as a danger signal for autoimmune diseases, 142 cites. Frontiers in immunology. 2017 May 23;8:598. doi: 10.3389/fimmu.2017.00598

11. Teng Y, Ren Y, Sayed M, Hu X, Lei C, Kumar A, Hutchins E, Mu J, Deng Z, Luo C, Sundaram K. Plant- 365
derived exosomal microRNAs shape the gut microbiota, 52 cites. Cell host & microbe. 2018 Nov 14;24(5):637-52. DOI: 10.1016/j.chom.2018.10.001

12. "Our Results So Far". Web blog post. American Gut Project. www.Americangut.org

13. "Solutions4". Web podcast. www.solutions4products.myshopify.com

14. Wilkins LJ, Monga M, Miller AW. Defining Dysbiosis for a cluster of chronic diseases, 5 cites. Scientific reports. 2019 Sep 9;9(1):1-0.
15. "Dr. Shinya - Proven Method to Cleanse Colon". YouTube Post. Enagic Kangen Water.
16. Enagic Kangen Water YouTube Channel. 9 February. 2015. Web. 9 February. 2015.
17. Gholipour, B. "Exhaled Pounds: How Fat Leaves the Body". LiveScience. www.livescience.com
18. "Ectoderm". Web course post. Embryology. www.embryology.med.unsw.edu.au
19. Baxter NT, Schmidt AW, Venkataraman A, Kim KS, Waldron C, Schmidt TM. Dynamics of human gut microbiota and short-chain fatty acids in response to dietary interventions with three fermentable fibers, 51 cites. MBio. 2019 Feb 26;10(1):e02566-18. DOI: 10.1128/mBio.02566-18
20.Cavaleri F, Bashar E. Potential synergies of β-hydroxybutyrate and butyrate on the modulation of metabolism, inflammation, cognition, and general health, 15 cites. Journal of nutrition and metabolism. 2018;2018. doi: 10.1155/2018/7195760

Chapter 6

1. Cahill Jr GF, Veech RL. Ketoacids? Good medicine?, 188 cites. Transactions of the American clinical and climatological association. 2003;114:149.
366
2. "Wayne Dyer - Morning Ah Guided Meditation for Manifesting Afirmations". YouTube Post. postmodernjungle. postmodernjungle YouTube Channel. 15 January. 2015. Web. 15 January. 2015.
3. Kinma, T. Risoldi, Z. "Sublingual and Buccal Medication Administration". Web blog post.
4. Healthline. www.healthline.com
5. He H, Lu Y, Qi J, Zhu Q, Chen Z, Wu W. Adapting liposomes for oral drug delivery, 43 cites. Acta pharmaceutica sinica B. 2019 Jan 1;9(1):36-48. doi: 10.1016/j.apsb.2018.06.005
6. Steffen KT, Hatakka A, Hofrichter M. Degradation of humic acids by the litter- decomposing

basidiomycete Collybia dryophila, 157 cites. Appl.
Environ. Microbiol.. 2002 Jul 1;68(7):3442-8. DOI:
10.1128/AEM.68.7.3442-3448.2002
7. King A. BAD SCIENCE: Oil pulling, 2 cites. Bdj. 2018;
224: 470.
8. "Certainty Iin Uncertain Times". Web blog post.
Tony Robbins. www.tonyrobbins.com
9. Burhoe, Brian. "Which Nuts Are Alkaline Forming?".
Web blog post. OEL – OurEverydayLife.
www.oureverydaylife.com
10. Dix, M. Sethi, S. "What Is Hypochlorhydria?". Web
blog post. Healthline. www.healthline.com
11. "Ruben Ostrea - Dr Hiromi Shinya Colonoscopy
Kangen Diet". YouTube Post. Roben Ostrea. Roben
Ostrea YouTube Channel. 11 December. 2015. Web. 11
December. 2015.
12. "Dr Hiromi Shinya --Colon Cleanse Using Kangen
Water". YouTube Post. JC Lim. JC Lim YouTube
Channel. 11 June. 2011. Web. 11 June. 2011.
367
13. Berczi I. Walter cannon's "fight or flight response"–
"acute stress response.", 2 cites. University of
Manitoba. 2015.
14. "Parasympathetic nervous system". Web post.
Wikipedia – The free encyclopedia.
www.en.wikipedia.org
15. "The DEEPEST Healing Sleep | 3.2Hz Delta Brain
Waves | REM Sleep Music - Binaural Beats".
YouTube Post. SleepTube - Hypnotic Relaxation.
SleepTube - Hypnotic Relaxation YouTube Channel.
24 October. 2019. Web. 24 October. 2019.
16. "Fluoride". Web blog post. Healthy Choices.
www.healthychoices.co.uk

Chapter 7

1. Schneider, T van. "If you want it, you might get it.
The Reticular Activating System explained". Web
blog post. Medium. www.medium.com
2. "How To Create The Future You Want with Dr. Joe
Dispenza". YouTube Post. Aubrey Marcus. Aubrey
Marcus YouTube Post. 21 August. 2019. Web. 21

August. 2019.

3. Courchesne-Loyer A, Lowry CM, St-Pierre V, Vandenberghe C, Fortier M, Castellano CA, Wagner JR, Cunnane SC. Emulsification increases the acute ketogenic effect and bioavailability of medium-chain triglycerides in humans: protein, carbohydrate, and fat metabolism, 6 cites. Current developments in nutrition. 2017 Jul 1;1(7):e000851. doi.org/10.3945/cdn.117.000851

4. Veech RL. Ketone esters increase brown fat in mice and overcome insulin resistance in other tissues in the rat, 12 cites. Annals of the New York academy of sciences. 2013 Oct;1302(1).DOI: 10.1111/nyas.12222 368

5. "Dr. Volek & Dr. Phinney - Translating the Basic Science of Nutritional Ketosis & Keto- Adaptation". YouTube Post. Virta Health. Virta Health YouTube Channel. 31 October. 2018. Web. 31 October. 2018.

6. Gomez-Arbelaez D, Crujeiras AB, Castro AI, Martinez-Olmos MA, Canton A, Ordoñez- Mayan L, Sajoux I, Galban C, Bellido D, Casanueva FF. Resting metabolic rate of obese patients under very low calorie ketogenic diet, 14 cites. Nutrition & metabolism. 2018 Dec;15(1):18. doi: 10.1186/s12986-018-0249-z

7. "How many calories are in one gram of fat, carbohydrate, or protein?". Web post. USDA

8. National Agricultural Library. www.nal.usda.gov

9. Frtiz, E.P. "Weighing In On The Keto Diet". Web blog post. KEMIN. www.kemin.com

10. "Dr. Benjamin Bikman - 'Insulin vs. Ketones - The Battle for Brown Fat'". YouTube Post. Low Carb Down Under. Low Carb Down Under YouTube Channel. 17 March. 2017. Web. 17 March. 2017.

11. Manninen AH. Very-low-carbohydrate diets and preservation of muscle mass, 81 cites. Nutrition & metabolism. 2006 Dec;3(1):1-4. doi: 10.1186/1743-7075-3-9

12. Moon JY, Choi MH, Kim J. Metabolic profiling of cholesterol and sex steroid hormones to monitor urological diseases, 17 cites. Endocrine-related

cancer. 2016 Oct

13. 1;23(10):R455-67. doi: 10.1530/ERC-16-0285

14. "Fructose-induced Hepatic De Novo Lipogenesis in Adolescents With Obesity". Web post. NIH – US National Library of Medicine. www.clinicaltrials.gov

15. "How Caloric Reduction Wrecks your Metabolism – Calories Part VI". Web blog post.

369

16. The Fasting Method. www.thefastingmethod.com

17. Bettelheim FA, Brown WH, Campbell MK, Farrell SO, Torres O. Introduction to general, organic and biochemistry. Nelson Education; 2012.

18. Müller TD, Nogueiras R, Andermann ML, Andrews ZB, Anker SD, Argente J, Batterham RL, Benoit SC, Bowers CY, Broglio F, Casanueva FF. Ghrelin, 452 cites. Molecular metabolism. 2015 Jun 1;4(6):437-60. doi: 10.1016/j.molmet.2015.03.005

19. Fetters, A. "Can You Gain Muscle While Losing Weight?". Web blog post. U.S News & World Report. www.health.usnews.com

20. "Why Sugar Can Wreck Your Sex Drive". Web blog post. Cleveland Clinic – Health Essentials. www.health.clevelandclinic.org

Chapter 8

1. "How to Slow Aging (and even reverse it)". YouTube Post. Veritasium. Veritasium YouTube Channel. 14 December. 2019. Web. 14 December. 2019.

Bonus Chapter

1. "Diabetes IS Lactic Acidosis.". YouTube Post. Dr. Darren Schmidt, DC. Dr. Darren Schmidt, DC YouTube Channel. 17 September. 2016. Web. 17 September. 2016.

2. "Dr Jerry Tennant - pH and Voltage - "Healing is Voltage"". YouTube Post. HealthAbundance411. HealthAbundance411 YouTube Channel. 30 April. 2013. Web. 30 April. 2013.

3. Higgins, C. "Lactate and lactic acidosis". Web blog post. acutecaretesting.org. www.acutecaretesting.org

370

4. Wu, B. Weatherspoon, D. "What's to know about

hemorrhagic stroke?". Web blog post.

5. Medical News Today. www.medicalnewstoday.com

6. Lip GY, Clementy N, Pierre B, Boyer M, Fauchier L. The Impact of Associated Diabetic Retinopathy on Stroke and Severe Bleeding Risk in Diabetic Patients With Atrial Fibrillation: Th e Loire Valley Atrial Fibrillation Project, 18 cites. Chest. 2015 Apr 1;147(4):1103-10. doi.org/10.1378/chest.14-2096

7. Gawenda M, Brunkwall J. Ruptured abdominal aortic aneurysm: the state of play, 24 cites. Deutsches Ärzteblatt International. 2012 Oct;109(43):727. doi: 10.3238/arztebl.2012.0727

8. Sun S, Ji Y, Kersten S, Qi L. Mechanisms of inflammatory responses in obese adipose tissue, 260 cites. Annual review of nutrition. 2012 Aug 21;32:261-86. doi: 10.1146/annurev-nutr-071811-150623

9. Samadi, D B. "Inflammation: The Battle to the Death Inside Our Bodies". Web blog post.

6. Observer. www.observer.com

7. Hunter P. The inflammation theory of disease, 147 cites. EMBO reports. 2012 Nov 1;13(11):968-70. doi: 10.1038/embor.2012.142

8. "Fight Inflammation to Help Prevent Heart Disease". Web blog post. Johns Hopkins Medicine - Health – Wellness & Prevention. www.hopkinsmedicine.org

9. "Treating the Inflammation of Asthma". Web blog post. Cleveland Clinic. www.my.clevelandclinic.org

10. Coussens LM, Werb Z. Inflammation and cancer, 12693 cites. Nature. 2002 Dec;420(6917):860-7. doi: 10.1038/nature01322

371

11. De Miguel C, Rudemiller NP, Abais JM, Mattson DL. Inflammation and hypertension: new understandings and potential therapeutic targets, 76 cites. Current hypertension reports. 2015 Jan 1;17(1):507. doi: 10.1007/s11906-014-0507-z

12. Pahwa R, Jialal I. Chronic inflammation, 33 cites. InStatPearls [Internet] 2018 Oct 27. StatPearls Publishing.

13. "Dr. Jerry Tennant - "An Understanding of How the Body Works" Part 2 (1/5)". YouTube Post. Astral1911. Astral1911 YouTube Channel. 11 September. 2010. Web. 11 September. 2010.

14. Otto AM. Warburg effect (s)—a biographical sketch of Otto Warburg and his impacts on tumor metabolism, 65 cites. Cancer & metabolism. 2016 Dec;4(1):5. doi: 10.1186/s40170-016-0145-9

15. Volk WA. Basic microbiology, 123 cites. HarperCollins; 1992.

THANK YOU FOR READING MY BOOK!

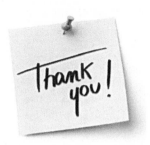

DOWNLOAD YOUR FREE GIFTS

Read This First

Just to say thanks for buying and reading my book, I would

like to give you a few free bonus gifts, no strings attached!

To Download Now, Visit:
http://www.drgregoketodoc.com/book-freegift

I appreciate your interest in my book, and I value your feedback as it helps me improve future versions of this book. I would appreciate it if you could leave your invaluable review on Amazon.com with your feedback. Thank you!

Made in the USA
Las Vegas, NV
30 January 2022

42661727R00187